The Final Diagnosis

The Final Diagnosis

What the Autopsy Reveals About Life and Death

Boris Datnow MD

and

Claire Datnow MA

Media Mint Publications
Birmingham, Alabama

FIRST MEDIA MINT BOOK EDITION, OCTOBER 2009

This is a work of nonfiction drawn from medical histories and autopsies. To protect the privacy of families and others involved, names of people and places have been changed, and specific details of events surrounding the case studies have been recreated or altered. Any resemblance to people living or dead is purely coincidental.
The Final Diagnosis: Copyright © 2009 by Boris Datnow and Claire Datnow. All rights reserved. No part of this book may be used or reproduced in any manner whatsoever without written permission except in the case of brief quotations embodied in critical articles or reviews.
For information:
Media Mint Publishers,
2021 Brae Trail,
Birmingham, Alabama 35242

www.mediamint.com

ISBN: 978-0-9842778-1-0

Book and Cover Design by Boris Datnow
Cover Photograph: Vigeland Park, Oslo, Norway
by Boris Datnow

Printed in the United States of America

Dedication

This book is dedicated to my children and their spouses Allen and Magos, Steve and Jacie, and Robyn and Stuart, and to my grandchildren, Sonia, Claudia, Emily, Lilly, Madeline and Elise, and to future generations to come. The work is also dedicated to the pursuit of excellence in medicine.

Table of Contents

Foreword

1 The Final Dialysis

2 A Case of Persistent Anemia

3 A Veteran of the Gulf War

4 Midnight Emergency

5 Sawdust Man

6 Death by Motorcycle?

7 Guilt by Transference

8 Denial

9 Double Indemnity

10 A Subtle Form of Neglect

11 The Homeless Rastafarian

12 Exhaustive Mania

13 A Case of Outrage

14 The Exhumation of Wiley Root

Future Diagnosis

Foreword

The death of a loved one is always painful, unsettling, frightening, and often quite mysterious. An autopsy explains the cause of death, and this often helps ease the anxiety that comes from not knowing or understanding why a loved one died. What is learned at autopsy can enhance the lives and, perhaps, the longevity of surviving family members.

As a pathologist, I perform clinical autopsies, or postmortem examinations. An autopsy is a medical procedure to determine a specific cause of death, and to learn about diseases or injuries that may be present. The autopsy provides insight into pathological processes and the factors that contributed to a patient's death, as well as information about the patient's health while living. Autopsies are performed to ensure the standard of care at hospitals. In addition, the autopsy can yield insight into how deaths can be prevented in the future. The most reliable and accurate way to diagnose the majority of diseases is still by direct examination of the organs at autopsy. It is a methodical anatomical investigation of the body and its organs by a trained physician

My medical specialty is Pathology. I chose to become a pathologist primarily because it is the most scientific branch of medicine, enabling the physician to track down and to locate the causes of an illness microscopically: to find its location, the pathological processes that occurred in the body, and the etiology of the disease. In addition, while working on a Bachelor of Science degree, I found that I thoroughly enjoyed working in the laboratory, indicating my predisposition for laboratory over clinical medicine.

There are several areas of specialization and sub-specialization within this field of medicine. The three main ones are, anatomic, clinical and forensic pathology. I am board certified in anatomic and clinical pathology. Anatomic pathology is the study of diseased tissue removed during surgery or at autopsy. Clinical pathology is the study of blood and its components, and the chemical testing of blood and body fluids for the purpose of assisting physicians with the diagnosis of disease. The Greek derivation of the word autopsy means to see for yourself. It is a specific medical procedure performed on a cadaver, by a trained physician.

I am fortunate to have received my general pathology training from the Mayo Clinic, Rochester, Minnesota. After earning a medical degree, a pathologist serves four years in residency studying the ways in which diseases affect the body and how they may result in death. This includes two years of anatomic pathology and two years of clinical pathology. The training for autopsy work is part of the residency in anatomic pathology. One year is devoted entirely to autopsies and the study of the organs. The training is done under the supervision of certified pathologists while performing actual autopsies. After residency training, the pathologist must pass an examination in order to be board certified by the College of American Pathologists.

A hospital pathologist performs autopsies to determine the disease or pathological process that caused death, and is limited to death by natural causes. When a patient dies in the hospital, with the permission of the next of kin, the hospital staff may order an autopsy to determine the cause of death. At one time hospitals were required to do an autopsy on all hospital deaths. Later this was modified to about ten percent; more recently autopsies are rarely performed except by special request from the medical staff.

When a patient expires in the hospital, a family member may request an autopsy, which was traditionally free of charge. Unfortunately, with tight budgets, most hospitals will no longer agree to this, and the family will be required to pay for the services of a hospital pathologist. The findings of a hospital's pathologist are intended to be independent, and in no way influenced by the clinicians that treated the patient. However, if the family prefers and can afford it, a private pathologist can be contracted. In that case, the autopsy may be done in a funeral home.

I am not a forensic pathologist, thus I do not perform autopsies on those who have died of unnatural causes—such as homicides, suicides, violent or suspicious accidents, drowning, crashes and shootings—where the cause of death may be a criminal matter. Forensic pathologists are public servants who work with government and law enforcement agencies and are employed by state and federal crime labs; in that capacity they have the use of state facilities. Forensic pathology is a sub specialty that studies unnatural causes of death as opposed to hospital pathology, where the emphasis is on finding natural causes of death. The forensic postmortem, which focuses on manner of death (gunshot wound, drowning, rape), is different to the autopsy, whose purpose is to discover the complex processes leading to natural deaths.

In most states a coroner is authorized to order an autopsy in the case of violent, traumatic deaths or other unnatural causes. A coroner is a political appointee, while a medical examiner is a physician, generally a pathologist with sub specialty training in forensic pathology. Autopsies can be ordered in every state when there is suspicion of wrongdoing. In addition, autopsies may be performed where there is a possible threat to public health, for example, epidemics, when etiology and exact nature of a disease is unknown, or there are concerns about the quality of health care. In the majority of states, an autopsy may also be performed if someone dies unattended by a physician or the attending physician is reluctant to sign the death certificate without an autopsy.

The coroner generally has the right to waive or limit the postmortem examination to an external exam or toxicology testing. However, if the family insists that an autopsy is needed, they may contact the coroner to explain their reasons for wanting an autopsy. If the coroner makes the decision not to order an autopsy, the family may arrange for a private autopsy.

Most religions permit autopsies. In the case of an orthodox Jew, a rabbi can be present at the autopsy. Moslems do not favor autopsies. It is best to seek the guidance of a religious counselor if there are any questions.

Before reading the case histories that follow, it would be helpful to understand the scientific protocol adhered to by the pathologist. First, in cases other than forensic, it is mandatory that the legal next-of-kin or responsible party, give signed permission authorizing the pathologist before he may perform an autopsy. Before beginning the autopsy, the body must be identified. Then the body is examined externally, and all abnormalities are noted: scars, blemishes, cuts and bruises. Much can be learned in this way. Routine measurements are also made, including the weight and length of the deceased.

Next, the internal organs are inspected. A Y-shaped incision is made from the shoulders to mid-chest, and into the pubic area. Because a cadaver has no blood pressure, there is little blood. An electric bone cutter in the shape of curved pruning shears is used to open the rib cage. A cut is made up each side of the rib cage, so that the chest plate, sternum, and the ribs are detached from rest of the skeleton. The chest plate is peeled off with the aid of a scalpel, which is used to dissect the soft tissues adhering to the chest plate. After the plate has been separated, the heart and lungs are exposed. The pericardial sac enclosing the heart is removed next. Each organ is carefully freed and removed for more detailed inspection.

The pathologist weighs the major organs—heart, lung, brain, kidney, liver, spleen—usually on a grocer's scale. The thyroid and adrenals, which are smaller, are weighed on a chemist's triple-beam balance. Any abnormalities on external or cut surfaces are noted, and then sliced and examined internally. Small pieces of abnormal areas, about the size of a postage stamp, are put in formalin, a fixative, for microscopic examination later.

To examine the brain, the skin is peeled back to uncover the skull bone. Then a bone saw is used to remove the cranium and expose the brain. The brain is usually suspended in fixative so that the dissection will be clean, neat, and accurate.

The pathologist returns all but the portions saved for analysis to the body cavity. Alternatively the organs may be cremated without being returned. The appropriate laws, and the wishes of the family are obeyed. To prepare for the funeral and embalming, the incisions are sutured, and the body is washed. The entire procedure takes 2 to 4 hours to complete.

The tissue, in preservative, is sent to the histology lab to be cut into thin sections for examination under the microscope before the pathologist writes up his final conclusions. The final report is sent out in under a month. All glass slides and tissue samples are retained. The pathologist correlates and interprets his findings, which are summarized in the autopsy report. The autopsy report has two parts: the Final Anatomic Diagnosis lists the disease processes in the order of their importance, beginning with the immediate cause of death followed by contributing causes. Incidental findings—which were not normal, but may or may not have contributed to the cause of death—are listed last. The second part of the report, the Final Statement, is an interpretation by the pathologist in a narrative format.

There are several reasons why a family may request an autopsy. An autopsy should be considered if there are concerns about the cause of death or the treatment the patient received. It provides the family with information that could prove useful to living members, for example, genetic or inheritable disorders. The autopsy could furnish key evidence if a family is planning litigation. Insurance companies may request an autopsy to settle claims—for example a cancer policy, an accidental death insurance rider, or double indemnity claims. Some physicians may request an autopsy to correlate their management and treatment of the patient with findings at autopsy. The possible underlying causes of death are numerous: a genetic flaw, age-related, fatal bacterial or virus infection, fatal damage by accident or violence, consumption of poisonous foods or overdose of drugs. Death occurs when the brain stops functioning due to lack of oxygen.

In rare instances a cause of death cannot be found and a conclusion of "no cause of death determined," issued. This is unsatisfactory, but a realistic fact.

Whatever the reasons for doing an autopsy, before making a decision it is wise for the family to contact a qualified pathologist to discuss any questions or concerns they may have. Where he deems it appropriate, the pathologist may suggest only a partial autopsy bearing on the suspected cause of death, in place of a complete procedure requiring dissection of the brain and all organs of the abdominal and thoracic cavity. Once the family has authorized an autopsy they may have additional questions. The most frequently asked questions are:

Will the autopsy interfere with the funeral? An autopsy should not postpone funeral services. The autopsy can be performed after the funeral service.

Can there be an open casket funeral? An autopsy can be performed after the body has been embalmed. An open-casket funeral can be held after the autopsy because the techniques of dissection do not disfigure the face. The pathologist performs the autopsy in a way that gives the appearance of an intact body suitable for showing in an open casket.

Is the autopsy covered by private insurance, Medicare or Medicaid? No, it is not.

I am often asked how I deal with the gory side of my work. I focus my attention on what I have been trained to do as a pathologist; I am spared the suffering and anguish of the terminally ill, and the heartache of the grieving relatives they leave behind. The nearest I come to feeling emotional distress is through empathy with the relatives of the dead, especially when I interview them.

In my opinion, the study of pathology is the most concrete and exact branch of medicine. Even though the law does not require that I do autopsies, there is almost always something significant for the family to learn. Often the autopsy reveals that the deceased suffered from an undiagnosed disease during life. Giving families the explanations they need is satisfying to me. It is also fulfilling as a physician to study the disease process in ways that may help to advance medical understanding.

The case histories that follow are based on actual autopsies performed over a period of more than thirty years. They reflect the prevailing statistics that the most common natural causes of death are heart attack, stroke and cancer. However, I have selected the most interesting cases, which may lead you to believe that non-forensic autopsies are often motivated by legal considerations. In fact, few non-forensic autopsies result in lawsuits. Having said that, human nature being what it is, there is an element of greed, even revenge that sometimes motivates the family of the deceased to request autopsies. There also are instances in which the family refused to accept the pathologist's conclusions as to the cause of death because of dogged ignorance or misplaced anger. In addition, the small sample of cases may give the impression of a higher percentage of major diagnostic errors than actually occur; however, studies of contemporary United States institutions indicate about 20% to 30% of autopsies detect diagnostic errors. Furthermore, more than a quarter of autopsies revealed a major unexpected discovery other than the primary cause of death, in other words, findings that would not have changed treatment, but may be important to the family and physician in the future.

While autopsies are among the most reliable methods of validating clinical diagnoses they have been steadily declining. In the 1940s, the rate of autopsies was about 50%. By the mid-1980s, the rate had dropped to between 10% and 15%. The reasons for the decline include the fact that autopsies are costly and not reimbursable, too heavy reliance on modern technology such as MRI and CAT scans, and the hospitals' fears of litigation.

The following chapters tell the human and medical stories behind autopsy cases. Like a good mystery, each one is salted with clues to assist the reader in deducing the final cause of death, revealed only at the end. I hope you will find the case histories intriguing, that they will reward you with new insights about the causes of death and how they relate to those dear to you.

1

The Final Dialysis

My task in the case of sixteen-year-old Renee Conroy was to find a cause of death, not to pass a legal opinion—that decision is the responsibility of the legal system. Yet my findings often provide key evidence that may be used by lawyers on either side of the case. Renee's parent came to me not solely for legal reasons; as part of the processes of grieving, they needed to understand what had claimed the life of their beloved daughter.

The day before her appointment for her routine dialysis, Renee Conroy came into the local ER complaining of lower abdominal pain. After examining her, the doctor prescribed

Butorphanol, a class four narcotic for relieving pain, and then transferred her to West End, a regional hospital, where she was admitted for observation.

The next day, Renee felt better and they proceeded with the scheduled dialysis. As Nurse Paton hooked Renee up to the machines, she noted that the patient was diminutive, with green eyes too large for her face, and a mane of red hair that seemed too heavy for her slender neck. About ten minutes into dialysis, Renee began complaining of severe abdominal pain, and the nurse administered a dose of Butorphanol.

The familiar routine of the dialysis unit, usually soothed the patients hooked up to dialysis machines, or artificial kidney apparatus, through slim tubes in their forearms. They relaxed in the steady hiss of fluids being exchanged, the blue glare of computer monitors, the pervasive smell of disinfectant and floor wax. Yet it was an impersonal place, designed for out patients who left nothing behind, not even memories of their fears and suffering, or their hopes and dreams.

Two hours into Renee's dialysis procedure, Nurse Paton glanced up from the nurses' station, observed that Renee was sleeping comfortably in a recliner, and made a note on her chart that the painkiller she had administered earlier was still in effect.

Satisfied that all was in order, Nurse Paton brought the paperwork up to date. When she next looked up, Renee was slumped over in her chair. Her arms hung limply, the magazine she had been flipping though had fallen to the floor. Nurse Paton hurried over to check Renee's vital signs, noting the saliva dribbling from the corner of her mouth, the bluish tint to her lips, and her clammy skin. Her heart rate registered at 145, and her blood pressure 156/104, indicating that her heart was racing above normal levels. The nurse immediately called a code blue over the intercom, and began emergency resuscitation. Within seconds, the emergency team arrived and took over as efficiently as a well-oiled engine. The team intubated Renee by inserting a breathing tube into her trachea, and hooked her up to a ventilator—an automatic breathing machine. After that they put up an IV to administer drugs to bring her blood pressure and heart rate to normal levels.

  The nurse shook the girl's thin shoulders and called insistently, "Renee, can you hear me? Renee, wake up!" She did not respond. Nurse Paton squeezed her limp hand gently, then more firmly, willing her to respond as she repeated, "Renee, can you hear me? Renee, wake up!" An IV dose of Narcan, a brain stimulant, failed to arouse the patient. Dr. Driscol, on duty in the ER, did a neurological assessment, observing that Renee's pupils were fixed and dilated, a sure indication of brain damage. He ordered the nurse to page Dr. Kilgore, the physician in charge of the dialysis unit.

Within minutes, Dr. Kilgore arrived and questioned Nurse Paton. He scanned Renee's medical chart and noted that she had been admitted to the emergency room at West End Hospital with a urinary tract infection the day before, and placed on a broad-spectrum antibiotic. He then ordered a Computed Tomography (CT) scan, or three-dimensional image, of Renee's brain and abdomen.

By this time Renee's parents, Andy and Mary Conroy had been alerted, and were waiting apprehensively by their daughter's bedside. Doctor Kilgore told them that the brain scan revealed no definite acute intra-cranial pathology. The abdominal scan showed a decreasing mass in the left ovary and left fallopian tube, compatible with a resolving tube-ovarian abscess. He went on to explain that the CT did not detect any tumors, hemorrhages, or blood clots in her brain. Mrs. Conroy's prayed that this was just one more crisis for their daughter to surmount.

Renee had been diagnosed with polycystic kidney disease (PKD) at age seven. The doctors had explained that polycystic kidney disease is a life-threatening genetic disorder, and affects more than 600,000 Americans and an estimated 12.5 million people worldwide—regardless of sex, age, race or ethnic origin. The disease causes multiple cysts on each kidney. These cysts grow and multiply, eventually causing the kidneys to shut down.

Dialysis and transplantation are the only known treatment methods for end-stage renal disease, or ESRD.

As predicted, Renee's kidneys steadily lost renal function; despite this, there were months that she felt well enough to attend school, where she made friends and achieved good grades. By the age of ten, all renal function ceased, requiring her to be put on continuous ambulatory peritoneal dialysis (CAD), a dialysate fluid that filtered waste from her body via a catheter.

A few months after her tenth birthday, Renee underwent a kidney transplant. To prevent rejection, routine immunosuppressive, or anti-rejection medications, were administered. Doctor Denton, her nephrologist, or specialist in kidney disease, advised them that Renee needed to stay on these drugs for the rest of her life. Nevertheless, Renee suffered an acute transplant rejection. To save her life, she had to come in for dialysis three times a week.

Now Renee lay in a coma on life support; still the Conroys refused to give up hope. They called Doctor Denton for a consultation. After examining Renee, Doctor Denton ordered an electroencephalogram (EEG), to measure the electrical activity in her brain. For the next four days, Dr. Denton continued monitoring Renee's brain function. The first EEG showed no electrical activity in the brain. The EEG test remained unchanged on the second day. A third EEG revealed increased intra-cranial pressure, an ominous sign that Renee's brain was beginning to swell. On the fourth day, a nuclear brain scan showed lack of blood flow in the cerebral arteries and venous sinuses, indicating irreversible brain damage.

Dr. Denton discussed the grim prognosis with the Conroys. He explained that as a result of complete brain death, there was no hope of their daughter recovering. However, she could be maintained on life support if they choose that option. The Conroys elected to maintain their daughter on life support; it was too soon for them to give up hope. A nasogastric feeding tube inserted into Renee's stomach provided liquid nourishment. She continued to receive dialysis and antibiotics to bring down a persistent fever. Renee's blood cultures were negative indicating that the infection in her urinary tract was not spreading.

As they held vigil at their daughter's bedside, the Conroys began to question the events preceding her coma. What happened in the dialysis unit in the crucial minutes that she had stopped breathing? Had she been monitored closely enough? Had she been given an overdose of Butorphanol (in patients with renal disease only a half dose should be used)? Was the use of Butorphanol appropriate under the circumstances? Had the doctor missed something seriously wrong with Renee when she had been admitted to the emergency room doubled over with abdominal pain?

Watching Renee laying inert and unresponsive to their loving words, Mr. Conroy felt his rage rising. A former marine, now an FBI agent, it was against his nature to stand by passively. Would a malpractice suit punish those who had done wrong? Mr. Conroy decided to contact the law firm of Poe, King and Rice, known for their success with medical malpractice cases.

After listening to Mr. Conroy's account of what had happened to his daughter, the attorney indicated that there might be a viable case for suing the hospital, the doctors, and other responsible parties. If Mr. Conroy choose to terminate life support and to sue the hospital, it would be wise to make arrangements for an autopsy by an independent pathologist. The pathologist's conclusions as to the cause of death would be key evidence in supporting the claim of malpractice and negligence.

The attorney advised Mr. Conroy that that an autopsy would be expensive. However, after the firm had gathered more information, he said that it was possible that they would consider picking up the cost on contingency. The attorney ended the conversation by recommending my services as an independent pathologist.

Mr. Conroy began by asking me if I was licensed by the state to do autopsies, and if I had any relationship to the hospital or its doctors. I reassured him that I was licensed, and that I had no affiliations to the hospital or its staff. I asked him to tell me about Renee, and the circumstances surrounding her going into coma. When he had finished, I advised him that my discoveries might or might not be helpful to his litigation, because the autopsy is an unbiased medical investigation, and that I would report my actual findings only.

As I listened to Mr. Conroy's somewhat rambling account of the events preceding Renee being put on life support, I began mentally sorting out the most salient information. The possibility that renal disease, or dialysis were causes of death seemed unlikely, since Renee had slipped into a coma so suddenly. A patient with end stage renal disease can be maintained on dialysis indefinitely. Her severe abdominal pain could have been acute peritonitis. My examination would pinpoint the exact origin of the peritonitis— ruptured appendix, perforated bowel, diverticulitis, ruptured bladder, or a perforated gastric ulcer. The brain would need to be examined as well. I am careful not to rule out any possibilities as this stage, as the autopsy might reveal something unexpected.

Mr. Conroy wanted to know if the autopsy would prove negligence on the part of the hospital. I explained that an autopsy is a scientific investigation to determine a cause of death, and that he should think of it as a special type of surgical procedure. The findings would reveal Renee's state of health while alive as well as why she died. These results could be used in court as evidence, and I would be available to testify as an expert witness if called on to do so. However, I could make no conclusions of negligence on the part of the hospital or the staff, as that would be a legal issue. I told Mr. Conroy that if he should decide to do an autopsy I would need a day's notice to make the necessary arrangements.

During the course of another long day at Renee's side, Mr. Conroy related the conversations with the lawyer and with me to his wife. The possibility of suing those responsible for Renee's misery provided little comfort for the parents faced with an irrevocable decision on whether to maintain their daughter on life support.

On the eighth day of Renee's coma, the Conroys met with the hospital's medical ethicist, Dr. Morales, a tall woman in her fifties, with gentle lemur-like eyes magnified by wire-rimmed glasses. She said that in their state, the law permits removal of food and water if a patient's condition is terminal and incurable, or if the patient is in a persistent vegetative state. Even if it caused distress, the medical ethicist knew that it was important for them to hear the truth; the doctors had pronounced Renee brain dead, and although she felt no pain, they had to consider the quality of her life. She reassured the Conroys that they did not have to make an immediate decision, and that they should take time to consider everything, including the enormous financial resources needed to keep Renee on life support.

Mr. Conroy's questions to Dr. Morales betrayed his anguish: Would taking Renee off life support be an act of mercy? A medical decision? A murder? Or just financial expediency?

The doctor replied that in her judgment as a medical ethicist, Renee's brain has died therefore her body had died. By removing life support they would allow their daughter to die with dignity, and with her family by her bedside.

"In other words, an act of mercy?"

"Yes, that is my opinion. But you and your wife are the only ones who can make the final decision."

After the medical ethicist left, the Conroys sat in a daze. Could they summon the strength to sign the document giving the hospital permission to remove Renee from life support? Even though the situation seemed hopeless, they clung to a belief that a miraculously a device or event would materialize, to put an end to their awful dilemma. Mr. Conroy paced the hospital corridors late at night, glancing into the rooms where patients slept restlessly. He returned his daughter's bedside to watch her sleeping as though dead, and something turned inside him. He told his wife that he was willing to take full responsibility for doing what needed to be done, if she would allow him to.

Nine days after Renee went into a coma, they suspended dialysis and took Renee off the ventilator. Prior to that, Mr. Conroy had signed a document directing the hospital not to take any heroic measures in the event of cardiopulmonary arrest. After about fifteen minutes, Renee became asystolic, or her heart stopped beating, and she was pronounced dead.

Mr. Conroy called me to arrange for an autopsy at the funeral home early the next morning. On arriving at the home, I introduced myself to the Conroys, waiting for me in a private room.

Glancing apprehensively at his wife sitting with her hands folded in her lap, Mr. Conroy asked, "Doctor, will it be alright to have an open casket showing after the autopsy?"

"When I have completed the autopsy, everything will be preserved and intact and will not interfere with your open showing," I reassured them.

"Thank you, Doctor," Mrs. Conroy responded.

I placed the authorization form on the desk. Putting on his glasses, Mr. Conroy scanned its contents, rereading the last paragraph authorizing me to remove and retain those organs and tissues needed for further analysis. He scrawled his signature on the bottom line, and the receptionist signed as a witness. As I was leaving, the Conroys asked how long it would take to complete the autopsy, and if I could give them a preliminary report after the autopsy that day. I told them that it would take us about three hours, and that I preferred not to give a report until I had time to look at the slides, analyze the results, and review the entire case. I would send them my final report in about ten days.

In the prep room, I found Duane Green, my diener, or assistant, waiting for me in his surgical scrubs. He had removed the body from the cooler and placed it on the autopsy table by means of a well-placed combination of pushes and shoves. After the body was positioned, Duane placed a "body block" under the patient's back. This rubber or plastic brick-shaped appliance causes the chest to protrude outward and the arms and neck to fall back, allowing the maximum exposure of the trunk for the incisions.

"Morning, Doc. I got everything ready to go," he greeted me, and I acknowledged his greeting. Wiry and strong, yet barely making five foot six, Duane appeared even shorter in shapeless, green surgical scrubs. Self-conscious of his height, he held his back ramrod straight like a soldier at attention. His cocoa skin glistened under the hot glare of ceiling lights.

It is not our custom to indulge in idle chatter when we are engaged in a scientific investigation to discover the cause of death. As I pulled on my scrubs, latex gloves and goggles, I registered the details of the room's interior: the spotless stainless-steel countertops, polished glass-fronted cabinets housing embalming materials, and cleanly scrubbed linoleum tiles. Just off center of the room, stood a gently sloping aluminum prep table, plumbed for running water, with spigots and faucets, to wash away blood and body fluids. Under a disposable white sheet I could discern the outline of a body. At the foot of the table stood a dissecting block on which Duane had set up assorted instruments—scissors, knives, forceps, needles, saws, and scalpels. On the counter, ready for use, stood a hanging scale, and labeled plastic containers filled with formaldehyde

I lifted one corner of the sheet and pulled it away to expose the body. With a stab of recognition, I noticed that Renee's bright red hair and freckled skin were exactly like her mother's. Reaching for my clipboard with a standard autopsy form attached to it, I began the external examination. I verified the body as that of Renee Conroy from the hospital wristband still attached to her corpse. Next, I filled in the date, case number, age, race and sex. Continuing the external examination, Duane measured and called out the length and estimated weight of the deceased for me to record. I made note of the nasogastric tube inserted through the nose, down the esophagus and into the stomach, and endotracheal tube inserted through the mouth into the windpipe, the portal shunt in the right forearm, and the Foley catheter into the bladder, as well as the precise length and location of healed scars on the abdomen and forearms. I marked these features on an outline drawing of the body. Duane then turned the body over. I could detect no visible abnormalities or injuries there.

Taking up my scalpel, I began the autopsy. I cut a classic Y-shaped incision from the shoulders down through the chest to the pubic bone. Then I carefully pulled back the skin, muscle, and soft tissues with a scalpel. I used an electric saw or bone cutter that has the appearance of curved pruning shears to open the ribcage. In this way I gained access to the organs of the thoracic and abdominal cavities. My diener held the tissue aside to expose the vital organs while I dissected the abdominal muscle away from the bottom of the rib cage and diaphragm in order to open the abdomen wider. The flaps of abdominal wall fell off to either side, and the abdominal organs were exposed. I methodically removed the heart, lungs, liver, spleen, and pancreas for examination, providing Duane with information about their size, texture, color, shape, and weight so that he could record it for me.

In addition to the routine examination of all organs, I focused my observations on the genito-unrinary system because of the patient's medical history. The right kidney could not be found as it had been removed surgically. The left kidney weighed only ten grams, whereas a normal kidney was about 75 grams. The kidney itself was tiny and scarred, with less than a centimeter of visible tissue present—a normal kidney is a smooth, shiny, bean-shaped organ about the size of a medium sized potato. Both ovaries, normally the size of a walnut, with a smooth and shiny white surface, were a dull greenish-gray, and covered with adherent, gooey, green pus, forming irregular blobs.

After weighing and measuring each organ, I inspected the outer surfaces for any abnormalities, and then dissected it for internal observation. After that, I selected tissue samples from suspicious areas, trimming them to about a centimeter and half. My diener placed these in a container of formalin to be processed for microscopic examination. This tissue would be processed in the lab by the histotechnologist. The technician would embed the tissue in a paraffin block, and then cut sections (2 to 5 microns) with a microtome, or instrument used to slice tissue specimens into transparent, ultra-thin sections. Next the slice would be placed on a glass slide, the wax removed by organic solvent, and special stains applied to outline cellar detail. I would inspect the prepared slides under a microscope for infections—parasitic, mitotic, and bacterial—and for pathologically altered cellular structures.

Duane removed the body block from under the deceased's back and placed it under the head, elevating it as if it were cushioned on a pillow. With a scalpel, I made a deep incision from behind one ear, over the crown of the head to behind the other ear. The skin and the underlying soft tissue were now divided into a front flap and a rear flap, and these were peeled back to expose the skull bones. Using an electric saw I cut through the skull, and removed the skull top, or calvarium, to expose the brain. I carefully removed the brain from the cavity by severing the cranial nerves and spinal cord, then lifted it out and placed it on the dissecting table. The soft tissue of the brain can easily be deformed; I therefore did not examine it during autopsy. Instead, my diener suspended the organ with string in a large jar of formalin to prevent it from sinking to the bottom and flattening out. The brain would remain in the jar for two weeks to "fix" or firm up the tissue so that I could later examine it without deforming it.

I replaced the bone and scalp with the hair so that the incisions on the scalp could not be detected. The face and the skin of the forehead were not disturbed.

After completing the autopsy, I pulled off the goggles, peeled off the gloves, removed the scrubs, and tossed them into a biohazard bag. I washed up in the adjacent washroom, leaving Duane to return the organs to the body cavity and close the incisions with a neat, baseball-type running suture.

I washed up, before completing my notes in an adjacent office. Thus far, the autopsy revealed that Renee's major organs were normal except for the brain and genitourinary system. There were bilateral tube-ovarian abscesses and evidence of a purulent cystitis. The polycystic kidneys and rejected kidney were present.

The brain was soft and partially liquefied, indicating prolonged brain necrosis, or death of cells.

On my way out, I collected the plastic containers to take back to the lab, poked my head into the funeral director's office to say goodbye, and drove back to my lab.

Three days later, the tissue slides prepared in the lab were ready for microscopic examination. The examination under the microscope confirmed the gross impressions I observed during the autopsy. I dictated a detailed report for my secretary to type up and mail to the Conroy family.

When he received the report, Mr. Conroy read it over carefully. After attempting to understand the medical terminology, he arranged to meet me for further explanation. From prior experience I know that it is difficult for the layperson to understand complex medical anatomy and physiology, and unfamiliar medical jargon, so I do my best to explain things as clearly as possible.

I asked Mr. Conroy to keep the report in front of him as I clarified it. First, I asked him to turn to the page headed, Final Anatomic Diagnoses. I waited for him to find the page then began reading, "'Point one: Ischemic necrosis of the brain secondary to prolonged anoxia. This shows that as a result of lack of oxygen to the brain, the brain tissues died."

"In other words Renee stopped breathing, so her brain was starved of oxygen?"

"That's correct. Over the course of several days her brain liquefied, turning to the consistency of oatmeal porridge with no identifiable structures."

"That shows that her brain tissue had died?" he asked.

"Correct. Now, point two reads: 'End stage renal atrophy, or withering away of the kidneys.' That's self explanatory."

"Yes, Renee had kidney disease from childhood."

"Point three: 'Bilateral lower lobe atelectasis. And point four: 'Terminal acute pulmonary edema and congestion.' Atelectasis is the medical term meaning her lungs were not aerated and filled with fluid as they would be in death."

I paused for questions then I read on. "Point five: 'Acute bilateral tube-ovarian abscesses.' And point six: 'Acute purulent cystitis.'"

"I knew it! My daughter suffered from bad ovarian abscesses and bad cystitis. That's why we took her to the emergency room. That's when they started her on the Butorphanol that ended up killing her!"

Although I suspected that the period of apnea, or halt in breathing, was induced by an overdose of Butorphanol, I said, "That's not a finding I can support in court. That's an inference."

"Why not?" the father demanded.

"Unfortunately, we can't test for Butorphanol nine days after its ingested."

"Well, the emergency physician's report and the discharge summary report state that she was given Butorphanol."

"Yes, that much is known. Now, let's go on to point seven: 'End stage renal disease on dialysis (clinical). And point eight: 'History of renal transplantation, transplant nephrectomy and rejection.'"

"I understand that part of the report. Renee was diagnosed with PKD. And she had a kidney transplant right after her tenth birthday, which was rejected and surgically removed."

"Yes, I read her medical records and they confirm that," I agreed, and then continued, "Point nine reads: 'Status post parathyroidectomy.' Having parathyroids removed is common in patients with renal disease. But don't concern yourself with that, it isn't important to understanding the cause of death. And point ten reads: 'Atherosclerosis aorta grade 1. Coronaries grade 1, Cerebrals grade 1.' This indicates that she had no heart related problems, as you would expect in a young woman."

"I am trying to understand it all . . . still I don't believe that she had to die."

"I know this is difficult for you. What is significant is that the final cause of death was prolonged anoxia, or lack of oxygen to the brain. In the autopsy report I state: 'The cause of death is cerebral, secondary to prolonged anoxia with necrosis of the brain. Cerebral anoxia occurred during dialysis following a dose of Butorphanol and an episode of supraventricular tachycardia. Additional findings include end stage renal disease, bilateral tube-ovarian abscess, and acute purulent cystitis.'"

"I want to ask you about the abscesses, Doctor."

"Go ahead."

"I read in your report that you found ovarian abscesses. But the hospital's clinical summary puzzles me, because it seems to contradict what you found." I heard him tuning the pages. "I'll read it to you, 'the abdominal CT showed decreasing mass in the left adnexa compatible with a resolving tube-ovarian abscess or scarring.' Does that mean the abscess was shrinking?"

"That was the radiologist's interpretation. However, at autopsy I found two large abscesses with inflammation on the surfaces, and that is the correct and final diagnosis. If you turn back to the sub-heading 'Genitourinary System' you will note that I found the ovaries embedded and surrounded by purulent fibrinous exudate, or clots of pus, forming bilateral tube-ovarian abscesses."

"Doctor, does that mean they misdiagnosed Renee's problem?"

From the results of the autopsy, it appeared that the radiologist and emergency doctor had failed to recognize the severity of Renee's condition. In my opinion, they should surgically have drained the abscesses before admitting her for dialysis. However, my role is to avoid making statements about the deceased's clinical management while alive, and to limit myself to my findings at autopsy.

"What I can say for certain is that I found two active abscesses in the abdomen," I replied, "But please understand that while this was a serious condition, it was not the cause of death."

"But," he insisted, "Do you think that I have grounds for a law suit?"

"I was not part of the clinical management of Renee's illness. It's up to the lawyers and a jury to make that determination."

Mr. Conroy requested that I send a copy of the autopsy report to his lawyer. I said I would, and asked him to call if he had any additional questions.

Shortly after this conversation, I received a letter stating that the law firm of Rice, Poe and King, representing the Conroys, had filed suit against West End Hospital and needed to take my deposition.

About a month later, Mr. Haskin, the defending attorney retained by the hospital, requested the paraffin blocks of the deceased's brain from which I had cut his slides. I was reluctant to lose custody of the original blocks, and as a compromise I offered to send unstained sections of brain to the defendant's pathologist.

A few days later, I received a letter from the defendant's law firm requesting additional unstained sections of tissue taken during the autopsy. I had no objection to this, and duly complied with the request.

Before the case went to court, Mr. King, the plaintiffs' lawyer, prepared his presentation. He interviewed the Conroys to get a family history, deposed the doctors and staff at West End Hospital, consulted with various specialists in the field, and held lengthy discussions with me.

In turn, the defendant's lawyer, Mr. Haskin, issued a subpoena for me to make a deposition before a court reporter— an officer duly authorized to administer oaths and swear in witnesses. I was asked to have the following items ready for examination.

1. Any and all tissue slides relating to the autopsy of Renee Conroy.

2. Any and all photographs relating to the autopsy.

3. Any or all correspondence with the Plaintiffs or their counsel.

I had these on hand the day of the deposition. The defendant's lawyer, Mr. King, Mr. Conroy and the court reporter were present.

During the deposition, proper legal procedure was assiduously followed. Mr. Haskin began by asking me to summarize my training and medical career. The lawyer probed me about any history of litigation, either personal or as a witness, hoping to uncover information that might discredit me as an expert witness. My answers were short and to the point. After this personal line of interrogation, Mr. Haskin went on to question me about the specific findings of the autopsy, hoping to cast doubt on my findings by focusing on anything that could be construed as vague, misleading, or suppositional. I have been involved in similar depositions, so the implied insults and insistent questions did not deter me. I patiently answered all questions as truthfully and plainly as I could. I made no statements about the nurses' or doctors' clinical management of Renee's case since I had not been party to it.

When the case came up for trial by jury, I was called to testify as an expert witness. After days of testimony and deliberations, the jury concluded that Renee had slipped into a deep sleep followed by apnea that resulted in brain death due to oxygen starvation. The jury further concluded that the Butorphanol was a contributing factor to inducing the apnea, or halt in breathing. The abscessed ovaries found at autopsy, indicated a missed opportunity for surgical intervention to drain the abscesses. In addition, more diligent monitoring of Renee's vital signs may have alerted attendants that she had stopped breathing, and CPU could have been administered in the vital minutes before brain death occurs; a period of only three to five minutes exists to get oxygen to the brain before irreversible damage sets in.

On the basis of negligence on the part of the dialysis unit, the attending physicians, and staff of West End Hospital, the jury awarded substantial damages to the Conroys. Still, the autopsy itself did not in itself prove negligence; it showed conclusively that the cause of death was cerebral, secondary to prolonged anoxia with necrosis of the brain, definitively ruling out any other cause of death.

In order to succeed in a claim for negligence, the claimant needs to prove that the doctor or other healthcare professional owed a duty to take care of the claimant and not to cause injury or harm. Medical negligence is a legal breach of duty of care owed to one person by another, which results in damage caused to that person. The Conroys were able to meet these legal standards, and thus were successful in their clinical negligence suit.

Nevertheless, a court cannot compel a hospital to change its practices or improve standards, it cannot discipline a health professional nor can it make them apologize; these actions can only be implemented by the hospital's own administration, or the state medical board. However, a finding of negligence and award of damages should compel a hospital and its insurers to review and improve its procedures.

2

A Case of Persistent Anemia

Despite technological advances such as CAT scanners, ultrasound and other sophisticated diagnostic equipment, studies suggest that a relatively high rate of misdiagnoses occurs; in almost half of these, a correct diagnosis would have resulted in a different, more effective treatment, as could have occurred in the case of Moses Dawkins.

Early on a Friday morning, the Mount Synod Emergency Medical Services received a distress call from the manager of the local NBC affiliate, alerting them that an employee, Moses Dawkins, a fifty-four year old videographer, had collapsed.

On that day, soon after Dawkins had checked in to work, the station received news of an explosion at a fertilizer plant on the outskirts of town. Dawkins—a big man with muscular arms, who had once been a football player—swung the heavy camera equipment onto his shoulder. As he headed out the door to cover the story, a wave of nausea overcame him. He bent over, clutched his stomach, vomited blood then slid to the floor saying that he was feeling weak.

Within minutes, the emergency team arrived to find Dawkins alert, but pale and clammy to the touch. His respiration was normal, but his blood pressure had fallen to 92/58, with a rapid, weak and thready pulse. He complained of stomach pain, nausea, and dizziness. Noting that Dawkins' vital signs were unstable, the paramedics contacted the Mount Synod Hospital and were instructed to start an IV line and transfuse Dawkins with 300ccs of normal saline, and then transport him to the hospital emergency room.

On arrival, Dawkins' condition had stabilized. He told Dr. Sheila Bressler, the attending emergency room physician, that he had been experiencing abdominal cramps, and black stools during the night. Nevertheless, he had decided to go to work, not wanting to miss more days than he had already missed that month due to a stomach ulcer. He added that the big football game was coming up on Saturday, and that he didn't want to cancel his assignment to video the game. Dr. Bressler said that she was a Bulldog fan, and she'd seen him at the games angling for the best shots. Concerned that Dawkins' skin and mucous membranes were markedly pale indicating blood loss, Dr. Bressler admitted him to the hospital for observation and gastrointestinal examination.

At this time Dr. Victor Potok, the internist treating Dawkins for the ulcer, was paged. Dr. Potok transfused four units of packed red blood cells into Dawkins; then scheduled an esophago-gastro-duodenoscopy (EGD), a colonoscopy, and a consult with Dr. Wyatt Jenkins, the surgeon who had examined Dawkins previously. After the transfusion, Dawkins said he felt better, and was taken for the EGD, or an examination of the lining of the esophagus, stomach and upper duodenum via a small camera on the end of a flexible tube inserted through the mouth

The results of the EGD indicated a healing duodenal ulcer. Doctors Potok and Jenkins attributed the improvement to the antibiotics they had prescribed.

Next, Dawkins was sedated and the fiber optic tube, used for colonoscopy examinations, inserted into his rectum and passed through to the ascending colon to examine the interior lining of the large intestine (rectum and colon). Unfortunately, there was so much blood in the area that the doctors could see very little. Dr. Jenkins made a differential diagnosis of a possible Mallory-Weiss tear, caused by the persistent vomiting, as a possible source of the bleeding. However, he cautioned Dr. Potok that other etiology, not yet detected, could be the source of the patient's hemorrhaging.

By now it was midday and the battery of tests had failed to pinpoint the location of Dawkins' bleeding. The doctors scheduled a Red Blood Cell (RBC) nuclear scan to find the exact site. Before Dawkins signed the permission form, they explained how the RBC worked. To prepare for the test, they would first inject a medication into his bloodstream that would "sensitize" the RBCs in his body, enabling them to be "tagged". About 20 minutes later, small amounts of radioactive material would be injected into a vein. He would then be asked to lie flat on a table while a special scanner detected the location and amount of radiation emitted by the tagged RBCs. The area showing the greatest concentration of RBCs would reveal the site of his bleeding.

While waiting for this test to be administered, the nurse on duty checked Dawkins' vital signs, and chatted with him about the up coming football game. The nurse noted on the chart that Dawkins seemed to be resting comfortably, sipping water and watching television over a period of about forty minutes. Then unexpectedly, Dawkins experienced shortness of breath and went into cardiac arrest. She immediately called a code blue then paged his attending physicians. Dr. Potok arrived within minutes; Dr. Jenkins was delayed by emergency surgery.

At that point, Dawkins' EKG showed some electrical activity in the heart, although he had no pulse. A blood transfusion was administered and Cardiopulmonary Resuscitation (CPR) started. Twenty minutes later, the doctor detected a pulse and Dawkins was transfused with additional blood. Despite these measures his blood pressure continued to drop and Dawkins' pulse was barely palpable, requiring immediate resumption of CPR. The team continued resuscitation for the next ten minutes; still no blood pressure could be palpated, and the pupils were now fixed and dilated. Nevertheless, the doctor ordered that they keep CPR going. Despite these resuscitation measures, the emergency team could not revive his pulse, his respiration, or any audible cardiac activity. Reluctantly, Dr. Potok instructed the team to discontinue resuscitation, and pronounced Dawkins dead. The family was then notified.

The circumstances surrounding Mr. Dawkins demise concerned and puzzled the doctors. This much was known: the patient had a history of peptic ulcers, colonic polyps, and chronic anemia. The records documented Dawkin's long history of bleeding from his GI tract. An EGD, done three weeks before, revealed a duodenal ulcer and esophagitis. To alleviate the ulcer, Dr. Potok started Dawkins on a fourteen-day regime of Biaxin and Prilosec. These medications appeared to have helped as the patient reported less discomfort. Despite these measures, Dawkins remained anemic, indicating that he was still actively bleeding from some source, and was given several additional transfusions.

A week prior to his death, Dawkins complained of feeling weak and exhausted. The EGD examination in the hospital, showed a healing duodenal ulcer. The colonoscopy was normal except for the scars where polyps had been removed from the sigmoid region. The day prior to his death, Dawkins had a complained of a bad sinking spell. The next day, the paramedics had been summoned to the TV station. While in the hospital undergoing tests, he had gone into cardiac arrest and died.

Why had the patient continued to bleed? Where was the source of the massive bleeding that killed him? Dr. Jenkins had made a differential diagnosis of a possible Mallory-Weiss tear as a result of persistent vomiting, but the EGD had not supported this finding. Dr. Jenkins's notes had cautioned that some other etiology could be at work.

The deceased's mother, Mrs. Lola Dawkins, refused to sign permission for a hospital autopsy, the most accurate method of finding a cause of death, as she was in a state of shock, and the thought of cutting into her son was distressing to her. Knowing how difficult it would be for Mrs. Dawkins to put her son to rest without a clear explanation why he had died, Mr. Benfield, the funeral director, suggested that she reconsider her refusal to do an autopsy. The findings would provide her with some peace of mind, he said, and would present family members with useful medical information.

When Mrs. Dawkins called, I reassured her that an autopsy is a scientific medical procedure, and that after the autopsy there can be a viewing by relatives and friends of the deceased. Later that day, I met with her to have her sign authorization for an autopsy.

Moses Dawkins' autopsy proceeded in a routine manner with the examination of the major organs. As he often did, Duane, my diener, asked from time to time, "Doc, have we found a cause of death yet?" I responded that I had not. While my diener had an adequate knowledge of anatomy, his knowledge of pathology was only rudimentary.

When I examined the stomach, however, I was struck by its unusual appearance. The organ was enlarged with thickened walls, and filled with fresh blood. After washing out the stomach, I opened it along the greater curvature, revealing that the interior lining had a distinctive cobblestone appearance. The diagnosis was unmistakable; I was looking at a case of Ménétrier's Disease, a rare syndrome characterized by prominent gastric folds and mucosal protein loss, for which no primary cause can be determined.

Next, I proceeded to look for ulcers but could find no evidence of any ulcerative disease. I completed my examination of the gastrointestinal tract (GI) and found no additional pathology there. The autopsy proved conclusively that the catastrophic bleed, which killed Dawkins, had originated in his stomach. Ménétrier's is a rare but curable condition. Had the doctors diagnosed Ménétrier's, they would have performed a total gastrectomy, or removal of the stomach, to save his life.

When Mrs. Dawkins received the autopsy report two weeks later, she tried to make sense of it. The report described each organ of the Moses' body—his heart, lungs, liver, spleen, G.I. tract, pancreas, adrenals, genitourinary system, thoracic and abdominal aorta, and brain. She read and reread the Final Anatomic Diagnosis, hoping to understand the case of death, but the medical jargon was too technical for her to decipher:

1. Massive upper gastrointestinal bleed with blood filling the stomach and proximal small bowel.

2. Chronic hypertrophic gastritis, or Ménétrier's Disease.

3. Left ventricular concentric hypertrophy (3.3cm).

4. Right ventricular hypertrophy and dilation (cor pulmonale).

5. Diffuse emphysematous bullae and anthracosis.

6. Chronic pleuritis.

7. Absence of left kidney, nephrectomy.

8. Hypertension (clinical).

9. Atherosclerosis, coronaries, grade 3 with calcification, aorta and cerebrals, diffuse, grade II.

She wondered how she missed noticing that her son had suffered from all these ailments. He was always so cheerful, and had a smile for everyone. She continued reading:

> Interpretation. The immediate cause of death is the massive upper gastro-intestinal bleed with a significant loss of circulating blood volume. The stomach has an interesting and characteristic pathology in the form of hypertrophic chronic gastritis (Ménétrier's Disease). In addition, there is moderate heart disease with left and right ventricular hypertrophy and coronary artery atherosclerosis. The lungs are extensively destroyed by advanced emphysema and anthracosis.

Mrs. Dawkins called me to discuss the autopsy report. In layman's terms I told her what is known about Ménétrier's Disease. Men between ages 30 and 60 are most likely to contract this rare disease. The illness causes giant folds of tissue to grow in the wall of the stomach. The tissue may become inflamed and may contain ulcers. The disease also causes loss of protein from the body. Ménétrier's increases the risk of stomach cancer. Case histories show it often results in massive gastric hemorrhaging. The autopsy showed that Moses Dawkins' circulating blood had been dumped into his stomach causing him to die of shock.

After a long pause while she absorbed all this information, Mrs. Dawkins asked if I thought that the doctors at Mount Synod Hospital knew what had been wrong with her son. I advised her to send copies of her son's hospital records to me, so that I could compare their diagnoses with my findings at autopsy. Ten days later, I to received a large brown envelope with the hospital records of Moses Dawkins. A cover letter from the law offices of Joyce R. Owens and Associates stated:

> Enclosed please find a copy of the medical records for Mr. Moses Dawkins on his last day at Mount Synod Hospital. You indicated that you wished to review the records to compare your findings at autopsy. Please contact our firm after you have completed your review.

In addition, there was a copy of the document in which Mrs. Dawkins gave the power of attorney to the firm, authorizing them to receive copies of the medical records of Moses Dawkins as well as myself. I speculated that Mrs. Dawkins was preparing to sue the hospital for malpractice.

I reviewed the records carefully, especially the EGD findings. Nowhere did they mention Ménétrier's Disease. In fact, Dawkins had been treated for a duodenal ulcer with conventional therapy. His physicians had failed to diagnose Menetriers as the cause of Mr. Dawkins persistent bleeding and chronic anemia. Yet I did not want to rush to judgment. While Ménétrier's is easy for a pathologist to see at autopsy, it is much more difficult to detect from an EGD. The disease is characterized by hypertrophic gastropathy (enlargement of the stomach lining with prominent folds and groves) giving it a characteristic cobblestone appearance. It is also associated with hypochlorhydria (low gastric acid production) and hypoprotenemia (due to protein leaching out through the affected mucosa). In adults the disease is usually chronic and severe enough to require subtotal gastrectomy (surgical removal of a large portion of the stomach). In addition, Ménétrier's Disease is rare—only about 200-300 cases worldwide per year. Dawkins' doctors had focused on more common causes of GI bleeding. However, because of their failure to control the bleeding and resultant persistent anemia, they should have opened Mr. Dawkins to examine him and to do a biopsy to rule out cancer. Had they done so, they would have seen his diseased stomach and removed it.

Before I made the call, I thought over what I would say to the attorney. As I have been trained to do, I did not make any statements about the clinical management of the patient, in which I had not been involved. I provided the attorney with the facts as revealed by the autopsy, avoiding a discussion of my opinion. I did acknowledge, however, that if the case went to trial in all probability the autopsy report together with other expert testimony, would indicate that the physicians had missed the diagnosis.

At the conclusion of our conversation, I consented to serve as an expert witness if called upon to do so. Months later, I heard that the Dawkins' case was settled out of court for an undisclosed sum, and never came to trial.

Autopsies remain a most reliable method of validating clinical diagnoses, yet as I have stated, the number performed has steadily declined. The reasons for the decline include the fact that autopsies are costly, over reliance on technology, and concern about litigation. Clearly, the autopsy can provide physicians with a valuable tool for prevention of unwitting repetition of misdiagnoses.

3

A Veteran of the Gulf War

The pulse, the urine, the sweat, all have sworn to say nothing, to give no indication, of any dangerous sicknesse. And yet I felle, that insensibly the disease prevailes.

John Donne

After decades of research, it was still unclear if the occurrence of Persian Gulf War Syndrome (GWS) or Persian Gulf War illness (GWI), reported by combat veterans of the 1991 Persian Gulf War, was higher than comparable populations, what the exact cause for the illness could be, or that it even existed. By the time I examined Sunny Malveaux on my table, he had been battling symptoms for many years, but was GWI the cause of death?

Sunny joined the Army National Guard; it helped pay for his college tuition, kept him physically fit, and made him feel like a real patriot. In reality, the drill weekends were mostly drudgery. Then, when he least expected it, he had been called to serve in the Persian Gulf War for six months.

He spent most of his tour traversing the alien moonscape of desert dunes eroded into grotesque shapes by violent sandstorms and blistering heat. When Malveaux returned from the Persian Gulf, he was declared fit to resume work. With boy-next-door good looks and a ready smile, he made an excellent salesman, rising through the ranks to become regional manger of a surgical supply company. Despite his success, Mrs. Malveaux noticed that her husband tired easily and was uncharacteristically irritable. He began complaining of joint aches, persistent headaches, stomach upsets, skin rashes, night sweats and difficulty sleeping. For a man in his late thirties these complaints seemed excessive and worrisome, and she insisted that he see a doctor.

In an attempt to find a satisfactory diagnosis for what ailed him, he visited several doctors. The physician would begin with an interview focusing on his medical history and present symptoms, and then proceed with a standard physical examination. Samples of blood and urine were sent to the laboratory for analysis. The physical exam revealed Malveaux to be a well-developed, well-nourished white male, with no abnormal vital signs. His lab tests read within the normal ranges. Since they could find nothing specifically wrong with him, the doctors made a wastebasket diagnosis of Post Stress Syndrome or Chronic Fatigue Syndrome. In truth, they didn't know what was causing his problems or how to treat them. They advised him to cut back on smoking, alcohol consumption, and fast food; he smoked two packs a day and consumed a six-pack of beer on weekends. Desperate to rid himself of these nagging symptoms, Malveaux reduced his smoking to a pack a day, his consumption of beer to two bottles a week, and avoided eating fast food. None of these changes noticeably improved his symptoms. In the interim, Malveaux continued to work and to participate in Army National Guard military exercises one weekend a month.

On these drills the men often reminisced about their experiences in the war, with one man's recollections triggering another. Malveaux joined in the bravado, although it evoked nasty images of bullet-ridden buildings, toxic oil-well fires, twisted corpses, SCUD alerts, and chemical warfare. In time, someone would tentatively mention that they suffered flu-like symptoms, which didn't seem to go away. Soon others chimed in with complaints about gastrointestinal problems, headaches, dizziness, joint pains and a host of other ailments for which there seemed to be no specific diagnosis. Those with no symptoms were skeptical, but others like Malveaux compared complaints and agreed it was weird, even scary not to know what was going on.

Malveaux's symptoms were cyclical; sometimes they worsened; at other times they improved. After two years, Malveaux's energy had not returned to the level it had been prior to the war. Although he considered talking to his unit commander, he decided against it fearing that he would come across as a hypochondriac. Not knowing where to turn next, Mrs. Malveaux called Terry Manheim, a close friend in The National Guard. Mr. Manheim told her that he and other vets were suffering from similar symptoms, causing rumors to circulate about the Gulf War Illness (GWI) that might explain what was wrong with them. Until recently, he had been unable to track down any specific information on the illness. He had all but given up hope when he heard about a Professor Sizemore, Chairman of Cancer Research at the University of Texas, doing research on GWI. For the past year he had been corresponding with the professor, and had received a letter that held out hope of treatment. Mrs. Malveaux asked Manheim to share all the information he had gathered thus far with her husband.

The letter from Professor Sizemore described not only his symptoms but also what was causing them. Malveaux read and reread the professor's letter with rising hope.

Dear Mr. Manheim,

After reading your letter, we would like to suggest from the symptoms you describe that you may be suffering from a microorganism infection called Mycoplasma fermentans (incognitos strain). This particular microorganism does not cross-react with tests for any of the 20+ Mycoplasmas, and routine laboratory blood tests do not detect this organism. One must employ a sensitive genetic marker analysis to detect this microorganism in biological samples. Even then it is difficult to find because it is found mainly inside cells in the body, not in body fluids. This particular Mycoplasma will cause chronic fatigue, recurrent fever, night sweats, joint pain, stomach upsets and cramps, headaches, skin rashes, heart pain, kidney pain, dizziness, nausea, and vision problems such as light sensitivity, blurred vision and floaters, hair loss, urination problems, eye pain, thyroid problems and, in extreme cases, paralysis. The good news is that unlike viruses, the mycoplasmas respond to the appropriate antibiotics. We have found that several courses of the antibiotic doxycycline work best, but it can take some time to recover from this infection. The majority of the medical community is relatively unaware of this disease, and those who are aware are likely to play down its possible role in illness, concentrating more on treating the peripheral symptoms of the syndrome. Since diagnosis may take some time, it may be of advantage to try a six-week cycle of doxycycline when the symptoms arise.

With Sizemore's letter in hand, Malveaux made an appointment to see Dr. Hazleton, who had been more sympathetic than the other physicians he had consulted.

Hazleton read Professor Sizemore's letter carefully, then said that he had read about this new illness in the medical journals. Still, he cautioned his patient that more research needed to be conducted before they could be certain of the findings. He recommended that Malveaux have a special blood test to confirm the presence of the Mycoplasma. In the meantime, a course of doxycycline couldn't do any harm. Dr. Hazelton warned him that patients often relapse after the first few cycles; however, subsequent relapses were generally milder, and most patients eventually recovered. The doctor explained that it would require a Gene Tracking test to identify this specific strain of Mycoplasma and to establish a specific link to GWI. At present, only Professor Sizemore conducted that particular test. Before Malveaux left that day, the nurse drew a blood sample to test for Mycoplasma. Malveaux felt like a drowning man grabbing a life jacket.

After several months on this regime, Manheim and Malveaux made the decision to share the information about GWI with the other soldiers on the next training weekend.

As the men relaxed before turning in for the night, they rambled on about Operation Desert Storm. Someone recommended a new book about Norman Schwarzkopf, another told about web sites popping up on the Internet airing opinions about the war. Then the talk turned to the bizarre symptoms some of the men had been experiencing, providing an opening for Manheim to share Sizemore's article. He could see the sudden kindling of hope in the men's eyes, when they heard about Mycoplasma and the treatment with doxycycline.

Malveaux told them that after a course of the antibiotic, he had more energy, the skin rash had disappeared, and he was sleeping more soundly. As forewarned, however, some symptoms reoccurred, in particular shortness of breath, chest pains and dizziness. Each time a course of dioxycycline had alleviated them.

Almost a year after Malveaux shared what he knew about GWI, the vets received a memo from the unit commander stating:

I feel it is my obligation to you and to the unit to make you aware of GWI so that you can be tested and treated for this infection.

There followed another memo providing information about where to apply for disability benefits. The war had been over for four years; now, when Malveaux had given up hope of official recognition of the illness, the unexpected had happened. The authorities were acknowledging GWI, even offering monthly monetary benefits to Gulf veterans with "significant symptoms that had defied conventional medical diagnosis." Compensation was to be based on proof of serious chronic disease or disability incurred during or aggravated by military service.

It took a while for Malveaux to track down and to obtain the necessary claim forms. Persian Gulf War veterans had to prove that their symptoms began within two years of leaving the Gulf area, which meant that he had to secure medical records from the doctors who had examined him. Ironically, a few months after he had sent in the copious paperwork, Veteran's Administration Secretary Brown changed this policy to allow Gulf War veterans a more realistic length of time to complete claim forms, while scientific research progressed on the causes of veterans' health problems.

In Malveaux's opinion, it was self-evident that he had contracted GWI, and that it was the cause of his problems. He resented having to fill in extensive forms as if his integrity were being questioned. After months of waiting, Malveaux's claim was approved. It was a relief to be included in the small percentage of veterans who would be receiving monetary benefits.

Although Malveaux continued to be productive, the fluctuations in his health were bothersome; he felt that he would never completely escape his illness. Two years passed in this fashion, then one day Malveaux collapsed at work. When he next opened his eyes he was dimly aware of the nurse applying a cold compress to his forehead. He had been dreaming of traversing the desert inside a tank, hearing the crump, crump, crump of artillery exploding around him.

After being treated for pneumonia with conventional antibiotics, Malveaux gradually improved and eventually resumed normal activity. He still insisted that the cause of his illness was GWI, although the doctors had diagnosed him with pneumonia, cautioning him that his chest X-rays showed a small spot on his right lung. They strongly advised him to come in for X-rays every six months to monitor any changes. Despite this, Malveaux remained convinced that all he needed to do when symptoms occurred was take antibiotics; as a result he did not come in for follow up X-rays.

After the first bout of pneumonia, another two years passed before he was admitted to the hospital. This time, he was dangerously ill. The doctors performed a thoracoscopy, a procedure that involves inserting a tube with a magnifying class and light on the end, into the pleural space to view his lungs, and also to biopsy the tissue for microscopic examination. The thoracoscopy revealed that the surface of the right lung was distorted, indicating an underlying tumor. His doctor advised Malveaux that if the biopsied tissue proved cancerous, he would need a thoracotomy to open his chest and to excise the tumor.

When the biopsy revealed the presence of cancerous cells, the surgeon performed a thoracotomy. Unfortunately, at that stage the cancer was inoperable. As a last resort, the doctors suggested a course of radiation and chemotherapy. Despite the grim prognosis, his family remained convinced that Malveaux was suffering from a severe recurrence of GWI. When Malveaux died eight days later, they held on to the belief that the GWI had killed him.

Malveaux's unit commander alerted Mrs. Malveaux that if her husband had died of lung cancer, the GWI benefits might cease. He recommended that she contact Art Findley, a lawyer working with GWI claims. Findley was familiar with the testimony of Professor Sizemore to the Committee on Veterans Affairs, and Subcommittee on Benefits of the United States House of

Representatives. He showed Mrs. Malveaux a transcript of Sizemore's testimony stating that he had been studying Gulf War Illnesses since 1993. It read:

The most troubling problem that veterans of Desert Storm face in trying to find adequate care for their illnesses is obtaining appropriate diagnosis and then adequate treatment. Most of the emphasis in diagnosing and treating GWI within the military and VA has been on stress-related conditions, such as Post Traumatic Stress Disorder. Since many patients do not fit this category, they usually receive an unknown illness diagnosis. This unfortunately results in their receiving reduced benefits.

Gulf War Illnesses (GWI) present as complex, multi-organ, chronic signs and symptoms that overlap with other chronic illnesses like Chronic Fatigue Syndrome (CFS), Fibromyalgia Syndrome (FMS) and Multiple Chemical Sensitivity Syndrome (MCSS). Unfortunately . . . the lack of clear-cut laboratory results in GWI cases tends to lend support for psychological or psychiatric diagnoses.

In the case of GWI, over 100,000 veterans of the Persian Gulf War of 1991, not including immediate family members, have been found to have this disorder. The variable incubation time of GWI, ranging from months to years, and the cyclic nature of the relapsing fevers and other signs and symptoms are consistent with diseases caused by biological and/or chemical or radiological agent(s).

The lawyer stated that Sizemore's testimony was key to Mrs. Malveaux's case for continuing to receive benefits. The Nicolson's testimony went on to say:

> It is time to put this war behind us, and treat the casualties and claims appropriately. Benefits and claims from the Persian Gulf War must be expanded to include immediate family members who have suffered and who continue to suffer because of veterans' illnesses that were transmitted to family members after the war.

To strengthen their claim, Findley advised Mrs. Malveaux to arrange for an autopsy, and I was called.

I obtained a history of the events prior to Malveaux's death from Mrs. Malveaux. She related that her husband, a veteran of the National Guard, had served in Desert Storm for approximately six months. Soon after returning, he complained of shortness of breath, frequent headaches, shoulder pains, general joint aches, and a host of other vague symptoms. Several doctors had examined him, but could not find what was making him sick.

Eventually tests revealed that he had Mycoplasma in his blood, which, she said, was linked to GWI. Malveaux was treated with antibiotics, which alleviated the symptoms, although they flared up from time to time. A week ago, he had been admitted to the hospital complaining of difficulty in breathing, and a high fever with chills. She stated that the doctor had opened his chest, but could not operate on her husband because he was too ill to survive the surgery. While she spoke, I jotted down notes. When she had finished, I asked exactly why the surgeons had opened Malveaux's chest, and what they had found there. Mrs. Malveaux became agitated and declared that she didn't know for sure; one doctor said he had cancer but another doctor said he did not. She stated that she didn't trust the doctors' diagnoses, as she knew for certain her husband had died of GWI.

I did not press for further information. From the wife's narrative, I suspected that her husband probably had inoperable lung cancer, but only the findings at autopsy would provide conclusive evidence.

In the course of the routine postmortem procedure, I observed that the right lung was not aerated, as a normal lung is light pink and has the consistency of a sponge; this lung was as red and solid as a steak. In addition, I found prominent, hard, white nodules scattered throughout beefy lung tissue. At the root of the lung, the lymph nodes were enlarged; when I cut in to them they were made up of the same hard, white tissue as the nodules, with the gritty consistency of an unripe pear, indicating that the tumor had spread to this area.

"Can you see how the cancer has spread through the lungs?" I asked Duane.

"Yeah, Doc, I think we've found a cause of death," he responded.

With my scalpel I cut and removed multiple tissue samples of the nodules, as well as samples from the affected lymph nodes. I placed these in preservative for processing in my laboratory, and examination under the microscope. Following this, all other organs were examined and I found no further evidence of the spread of cancer cells.

My final anatomic diagnoses revealed:

1. Poorly differentiated (grade 4) alveolar cell adenocarcinoma of the right lung with metastasis to the right hilar lymph nodes, and with secondary thrombosis of the right pulmonary artery.

2. Left lung with moderate emphysema and anthracosis.

3. Right acute pleuritis.

4. Post thoracoscopy and thoracotomy.

5. Atherosclerosis: coronaries grade 3, aorta grade 2, cerebrals grade 1.

Conclusion: The immediate cause of death is thrombosis of the right pulmonary artery with advanced alveolar cell adenocarcinoma in all the right lung lobes and with metastasis to the hilar lymph nodes.

As I had suspected, the deceased had advanced lung cancer, most likely smoking related. Before sending out my final report, however, I researched the latest findings on GWI to be certain that I had not missed any anatomical features associated with this illness. After perusing the current literature, it was apparent that the research was far from conclusive. Moreover, a heated and politicized debate about GWI was being waged. Many researchers claimed that GWI was an illness linked to a specific Mycoplasma, or a pathogenic microorganism, accusing those who denied it of taking part in a government cover up. Others contended that the research had failed to find a definitive cause for the symptoms veterans described, or proof that GWI even existed. My findings at autopsy revealed no evidence that Malveaux's death was linked to GWI.

Mrs. Malveaux and her lawyer were dissatisfied with my autopsy report. Her lawyer advised her to contact the

Veterans Benefits counselor at the nearest VA regional office for assistance. After months of fighting red tape, Mrs. Malveaux was granted continued benefits, but not nearly in the amount she felt entitled to.

Mrs. Malveaux became a crusader for Operation Desert Shield/Storm Association (ODSA), an organization lobbying to improve diagnosis, treatment and benefits for veterans of Desert Storm. She never acknowledged that her husband had died of lung cancer. I could not help surmising that his family's conviction that Malveaux suffered from GWI had prevented them from seeking appropriate treatment for cancer until it was too late. His case serves as a warning not to allow preconceptions or misconceptions to impair judgment that prevents an individual from receiving appropriate treatment in time.

4

Midnight Emergency

Rural hospitals face a number of challenges by virtue of their lack of staff and facilities, remote geographical location, higher number of uninsured patients, and shortage of community resources, factors often resulting in increased costs of running the hospitals. Despite the low volume of patients, small hospitals must offer all essential services, including emergency rooms, because they are the single provider of health care in the community. The circumstances surrounding the demise of Leroy Odum lead me to believe that he had received incompetent hospital care in his town of Oakville, but was this a direct cause of death?

Mr. Odum, the only mechanic in the village of Oakville, took ill on a blistering afternoon in late August. There isn't much to Oakville. The railroad tracks divide the main street into west and east, with an abandoned, wooden train depot at the west end, and Blountville County Hospital, a one-story yellow brick structure, at the east end. Up on the highway, Leroy's ramshackle filling station doubles as a grocery store and a café, serving cold drinks, beer and barbeque sandwiches. The local accent is spiced with a drawling nasal twang that takes awhile for strangers to decipher.

On the afternoon Mr. Odum became ill, he was working on a Chevy pickup truck. With a loud groan he unfolded his six foot three inches from under the hood then quickly doubled over with colicky pains in his stomach. When his daughter, Dolly Odum, rushed outside to help her father, he waved her away then leaned against the pickup and closed his eyes. The night before, Odum had experienced a bout of cramps and vomiting that he attributed to having eaten something that disagreed with him–now the pains had returned.

When the spasms eased, Odum straightened up, doused his face and neck with cold water, drying off with a clean rag. He asked Dolly to get him an ice-cold coke from the vending machine, slurped it down, and then went back to work despite her protests.

That evening at dinner, Odum said he was hungry, but after taking a few bites of a pork chop with mashed potatoes and gravy, he just pecked at the food on his plate. About an hour after dinner, he had another attack of cramps. To ease the pain, Dolly gave him an antacid tablet with a glass of warm milk. Around eleven o'clock, she was awakened by her father's loud groaning. She dressed hastily and drove him to Blountville County Hospital.

Dr. Gupta Rushdie, the doctor on call, was new to their small, closely-knit community. She noted on the chart that Odum had marked abdominal tenderness and thus questioned him about his drinking habits to rule out pancreatitis. Gallstones presented the other possible cause for the severe pain. After completing the case history without making a definitive diagnosis, Dr. Rushdie wrote: 'abdominal pain, probable severe gastritis, rule out pancreatitis and gall stones.' She ordered the patient to be admitted to the hospital for observation, prescribed Pepcid and Maalox for gastritis, Phenergan for nausea and vomiting, and as a routine supportive measure ordered an IV to keep the patient hydrated.

Over the next several hours the nurse on duty noted that the patient was awake, alert, oriented and resting comfortably. Later, he complained of constipation, requesting a laxative. The nurse notified the doctor who gave permission to administer the laxative. Soon afterwards, he had another bout of nausea and vomiting. After it passed, he dozed off and didn't seem to be in distress. The next morning, Mr. Odum ate a soft breakfast and bathed.

When Dolly came to visit, he assured her that he was feeling fine. He said that he hoped Dr. Rushdie would discharge him so that he could get back to work. At noon, he consumed a light lunch. When the doctor looked in on her patient, he appeared to be in no discomfort, and she instructed the nurse to remove the IV. Odum was discharged around three o'clock that day. Dr. Rushdie prescribed medications for two weeks, and suggested that Leroy make an appointment with his family practitioner the following week to check on his status.

That evening, Dolly and her boy friend, Jim Echols, watched a sitcom on television, while her father dozed in his recliner. Around ten o'clock he experienced an attack of severe abdominal pain. When Dolly called Blountville County Hospital to send an ambulance to their home on 145 Elm Street, the operator put her on hold despite her plea that her father needed urgent medical assistance. In desperation she hung up and called the police. They arrived at the house within minutes, to find Mr. Odum passed out on the floor and unresponsive. They advised her to transport the sick man to the hospital. With the assistance of the police, Jim carried Mr. Odum to his car and covered him with a blanket. Dolly sat in the back with her father. With red lights and siren going, Jim sped to the hospital, escorted by the police.

When they pulled up to emergency entrance, they were dismayed to find no one in attendance and the doors locked. The police knocked on the plate glass doors and shouted, "Open up! We have an emergency!" When no one came, Jim ran around the building to the front entrance where he found the night orderly sitting on the bench outside smoking.

"For God sake open the emergency room doors! There's a man dying."

The orderly muttered that he was unaware that the doors had been locked and hurried inside. When he unlocked the door and wheeled Odum into the emergency room, no pulse or respiration could be detected, his skin was cold and clammy, and his pupils were fixed and dilated. According to the hospital records, a code blue was called. The doctor on call arrived in the midst of intensive resuscitation proceedings known as CPR, or cardiopulmonary resuscitation by means of external cardiac massage and artificial mouth to mouth respiration to restore circulation of the blood and prevent death or brain damage due to lack of oxygen. When the CPR procedures failed to revive the patient, they were discontinued on the doctors' orders, and Odum was pronounced dead.

Family members arrived at the hospital at the first gray light of dawn, numb with shock, demanding to know why Leroy Odum had died so suddenly, and so soon after being released from the hospital.ABC Rushdie said that she would ask the hospital administrator, Ray Nesbitt, to do an autopsy to determine the exact cause of death.

Odum's niece, Betty Odum, who worked as a paralegal for the town's attorney David Spiegel, was determined to find out exactly what had happened to her uncle. Dolly told her that on August 20, her father had gone to the hospital emergency room complaining of severe abdominal pain, nausea and vomiting. He was admitted to the hospital for overnight observation then discharged the following day with instructions to make an appointment with his primary care physician. At home that evening, he had a relapse of the vomiting and pain. Around 11:00 P.M. Dolly told her cousin that she had called the ambulance service but was put on hold. She then called the police. With the police escort they drove to the hospital emergency room. When they arrived, no one was in attendance at the entrance, and the doors had been locked. Betty Odum called her boss, David Speigel. After hearing the extraordinary circumstances of Odum's death, Mr. Spiegel advised the family to authorize an autopsy as Dr. Rushdie had recommended. If the hospital agreed to the autopsy, they would bear the costs.

Betty Odum waited outside the hospital administrator's office until he arrived at work that morning. After listening to the history of what had happened to Roy Odum, Mr. Nesbitt informed her that the hospital did not have a pathologist on staff, and therefore could not perform the postmortem. The administrator expressed his regrets and condolences, and advised her to contact the funeral home to take possession of the body.

The paralegal related her conversation with the administrator to her boss, who then contacted me. Because the family could not afford to pay for the autopsy, Mr. Speigel agreed to cover the cost, as he believed that Roy Odum's case merited a lawsuit.

When the abdomen was exposed at autopsy, I observed that a loop of small bowel had a distinctly blue-black appearance in sharp contrast to the adjacent loops that were light pink and glistening. On closer inspection, the blue loop was friable, or crumbly, to the touch rather than soft and elastic. The affected loop was filled with blood and had twisted on itself, thus cutting off its blood supply, leading to necrosis, or premature tissue death. I also noted that the abdominal fluid, normally clear and watery, was tinged with blood. The other organs of the abdomen and chest cavity showed no additional pathology.

Ten days after the funeral, I mailed Mr. Spiegel my complete report. The attorney thought that he understood the gist of my findings enough to confirm his prior opinion. To be sure, he called me to clarify his interpretation of the autopsy finding. Only then did he call Betty Odum into his office.

Mr. Spiegel informed her that he had just received the autopsy report. He went on to explain that the autopsy had revealed an acute infarction, or a dead loop of the small bowel with secondary hemorrhagic ascites, or excessive blood-tinged fluid in the abdominal cavity. The hemorrhage resulted in shock and was the cause of death. The infarction of the small bowel was most likely due to a spontaneous volvulus, or twisting of the bowel, which cut off circulation. The findings revealed no history of previous abdominal surgery or peritoneal fibrous adhesions, or bowel abnormalities. Except for the pathology described, the pathologist had found no other pathologic abnormalities.

My report stated the medical facts only. In a follow-up interview with the attorney, however, I indicated that, in my judgment, Leroy Odum's death had been preventable, if he had received timely and appropriate surgical intervention to resect, or surgically remove, the dead bowel and then to reconnect the severed intestine. Based on these facts and opinions, Mr. Spiegel counseled the Odum family to proceed with a civil lawsuit.

At the opening of Mr. Odum's trial, the emergency room nurse on duty, Jane Singleton, was called to the stand. She said that she had worked at Blountville County Hospital for thirty years, starting as a nursing aide. When her husband, Reginald Singleton, passed away just a year ago, she decided to take the night shift because she was lonely, and because it paid more. Her duties as night nurse included taking care of the in-patients and those that arrived at the ER. The nurses' station was conveniently located adjacent to both the ward on the one side and the ER on the other.

At the time of Leroy Odums' arrival there were three patients in the ward: one elderly woman with malnutrition on an IV, a man in his fifties recovering from hernial surgery, and an aged patient recovering from pneumonia. None of these patients required intensive care. In fact, the hospital did not have an Intensive Care Unit. She had checked the patients' vital signs every two hours, noting the results on their charts. When questioned as to why the door had been locked, the nurse said she did it for security reasons, although she had not been authorized to do so. After lengthy cross-examination, the nurse admitted that she had gone to the cafeteria to retrieve dinner that a friend who worked in the kitchen had put aside for her. She stated that she had immediately started CPR and called Dr. Rushdie when Roy Odum had been wheeled into the emergency room.

Jackson Kelly, the orderly on duty at the time, was called to the stand after Nurse Singleton stepped down. Mr. Kelley testified that on the night of August 21, he had been taking a smoking break, when a man came tell him that the emergency room doors were locked. He had rushed to open them from inside. When asked why he had not heard the police hammering on the doors, he said that he was somewhat hard of hearing. He stated that he had not seen Nurse Singleton at the nursing station, maintaining under cross-examination that his attention had been focused on getting the doors open, and Mr. Odum onto the stretcher.

The hospital administrator, Mr. Nesbitt, served on the Blountville County Hospital's Board of Directors together with the mayor, bank manager, preacher, school superintendent, and owner of the town's most prosperous business. He stated that he had begun his career as a paramedic with an ambulance service in a nearby town. On cross-examination he acknowledged that he did not have a college degree directly related to his work as hospital administrator.

The attorney for the plaintiff waved an official-looking document before the administrator. "Mr. Nesbitt, isn't it a fact that the Joint Commission on the Accreditation of Heath Care

Organizations found that of 23 hospitals within a 50-mile radius of the city of Bington—the nearest large city with a population of one million in the greater metropolitan area—Blountville County Hospital ranked only 21st?"

Mr. Nesbitt shot back, "I do not want to minimize what happened to Mr. Odum, but I would appreciate the chance to put things in perspective." He cleared his throat and looked directly at the jury before continuing. "There are many factors that can affect statistical data, such as how ill the patients are, the type of medical procedures offered, and the number of serious trauma cases treated in an emergency room. Our hospital is connected to a 124-bed nursing home and ends up with more than its share of elderly, sick patients who are nearing the end. In a rural hospital such as ours with only thirty beds, a few deaths can easily skew its death rate."

"But isn't it true that your ER is understaffed to the extent that Nurse Singleton was absent when the police were pounding on the doors of the emergency room?"

Mr. Nesbitt responded, "In a town of about 6,000, the ER is under utilized. There are few violent crimes in our town—stabbings, gunshot wounds, overdosing on drugs, car accidents—which keep big city emergency rooms busy. And common medical emergencies like heart attacks, choking and acute abdomens occur on an infrequent basis. Nevertheless, in order to keep our license, the state and county require we maintain an emergency facility. Truth to tell, the need is not great, and an ER at a larger medical facility could better service the community."

"Are you saying that your hospital cannot adequately treat patients like Mr. Odum when they come to the ER in dire need?"

"No. I'm trying to explain that our hospital focuses on providing good basic care to its patients. But we're a rural hospital and do not have hi-tech equipment to do sophisticated procedures."

After that, Dr. Rushdie took the stand. Attorney Speigel for the plaintiffs wanted her to explain how she had diagnosed Mr. Odum's condition. Dr. Rushdie said that she had made a provisional diagnosis of severe gastritis. She had then ordered X-rays to rule out other possible causes. Being a small hospital, there was not a radiologist on the staff, and the X-rays were sent to a radiologist in Bington city hospital for interpretation. When she received the radiologist report two days later, it showed SB0, or a small bowel obstruction. Unfortunately, by then Mr. Odum was no longer alive.

Next, a surgeon was called to testify as an expert witness on behalf of the plaintiffs. He explained that small bowel obstruction refers to a blockage of the small intestine. Symptoms, which usually come on suddenly, are severe cramping, abdominal pain, abdominal bloating, nausea, vomiting and the absence of bowel movements. The most common causes of small intestinal obstruction are post-surgical abdominal adhesions (scarring from previous surgery) or hernias. Other less common causes include tumors and inflammatory conditions affecting the small intestine, such as Crohn's disease. Small bowel obstruction accounts for 5% of acute surgical emergencies: adhesions (60%), strangulated hernia, bowel trapped in the hernia that twists on itself (20%), malignancy, or tumors (5%), spontaneous volvulus, or twisting of the bowel (5%).

The diagnosis is usually made through X-ray imaging of the abdomen, which will show distended loops of small bowel without any air in the colon (large bowel). If the X-ray proves inconclusive, a CT scan may be performed to confirm the diagnosis.

The expert witness went on to say that the treatment for SBO typically involves hospitalizing patients to administer IV fluids. In addition to these supportive measures, a surgeon should be consulted to consider the need for surgical intervention. In many cases, the obstruction is partial and slowly resolves after supportive measures. However, in some cases, the obstruction worsens to the point that the blood supply to an area of bowel is jeopardized and emergency surgery becomes necessary.

In summation, the plaintiff's lawyer asserted that Mr. Odum had been discharged without a surgical consult, and the untreated obstruction had resulted in death. To make matters worse, the delay in starting CPR was due to extreme negligence on the part of the ambulance service and hospital emergency room.

The Odums were awarded a substantial settlement. Leroy Odum was a casualty of a series of mismanagements and mishaps, perpetrated without malice, which led to his untimely demise.

In my opinion, it is financially impractical for a small rural hospital to maintain 24-hour emergency service, seven days a week, effectively and efficiently. If required to maintain an ER by law, their hours of operation should be limited. Specific emergency contact numbers should be posted on the door for patients who arrive after hours. Local departments equipped to render emergency aid—such as ambulance, fire, and police services—should be aware of these hours of operation, and be on standby to transport patients to the nearest operating ER facility. In particular, an ambulance service staffed with paramedics who can administer drugs and perform life-saving procedures on the way to the hospital can save lives. A national emergency number, which can rapidly identify the calling number and street address, should be used in each state. In addition, dispatchers should require medical training so that they can give instructions while the patient waits for emergency medical services to arrive.

5

Sawdust Man

Seventy-five-year-old Woodrow Peel died while on the job he had held for over forty years. My findings at autopsy conclusively revealed the disease processes that had lead to Peel's death. In addition, my interview with Gladys Peel, his widow, served to corroborate my conclusion that if the deceased had recognized the gravity of his symptoms he might well had called 911 and saved his life.

Woodrow Peel's shift at the Boyse Sawmill, started at 3:00 p.m., when the sun had passed its zenith but the busy day was far from done; it ended at 2:00 a.m., when the moon began to wane, and the world dreamt on. At precisely 2:15 in the afternoon, he pulled on a cotton shirt and bib overalls that his wife Gladys had set out for him, tied a red bandana loosely around his neck, and shoved an old straw hat onto his head. In the kitchen he slurped down a mug of coffee, while his wife made sandwiches for him and her nephew. Lean and lanky, dark as midnight, with big hands that could hammer nails into the hardest wood, he ignored Gladys's muttering that it was time for him to retire because he came back from work exhausted and short of breath; he had already told her he would rather die on the job than be put out to pasture.

Stepping outside, Peel laced on his heavy work boots, standing at attention on the doormat like old soldiers, then lit a cigarette, noting that the first cool front of the fall has arrived to nose out the soggy summer heat. Around him the forest loomed darkly over the town like a wounded dragon shorn of its scales. In the 1980s, when the corporation came to town promising jobs and prosperity, the town's people greeted the company with open arms. Soon thereafter, Boyse began bulldozing roads through the forest for the logging trucks.

After walking the three miles to the Boyse Corporation sawmill, Peel arrived at exactly on time, punched his card into the time clock, then picked his way across the timber yard to the fuel house at the far end of the operation. As he trudged across the busy yard he enjoyed the familiar sensation of churned earth and sawdust yielding beneath his boots, the smell of newly cut timber tickling his nose, and the steady din of heavy machinery in his ears. Around him, timber in every stage of production waited to be processed and shipped to its destination. A felled forest of raw logs slid along conveyor belts toward the jaws of a debarking machine, then to the rotary saw to be sliced into planks. Smoking mounds of sawdust, scraped dirt and wood chips, neatly stacked rows of creosote-soaked crossties, tall palettes of low-grade lumber, and tons of furniture-grade hardwood oak and sweet gum waited for shipment to customers. "Hey, Sawdust Man," a big man called from his perch on a backhoe.

"Good mornin', Pete," Peel replied, tipping his straw hat.

Toward the back end of the yard Peel found his nephew, Jesse, loading air-dried timber into to the kilns for the final drying.

"Man, this work's too hard!" Jesse said.

"You still young and strong."

"Maybe so, but I ain't gonna break my back for nobody!"

Peel handed over Jesse's share of sandwiches from the lunch pail then continued to the sawdust shed adjacent to the boiler. Despite the cool spell, he felt much too hot, he had heartburn, and his stomach was queasy. The thought crossed his mind that maybe he was getting too old for this kind of work. But he'd worked from the day he left school, when he turned eleven, to help on the farm. He was habituated to work; it gave him a sense of purpose, a place to go in life. And he really derived satisfaction from his job. Given the opportunity to go to college he might have become an engineer; that's what Mr. Carver, the plant superintendent, said. Peel has an instinct for the workings of machinery and Mr. Carver has come to rely on him to fix mechanical glitches in the conveyor belt and boiler.

On reaching the shed, he put his lunch pail beneath an old palette he used as a chair, picked up a broom and began sweeping spilled sawdust towards the hopper. He had the job of making sure that the sawdust, collected on conveyer belts beneath the cutting saw, moved smoothly from the hopper into the boiler that fed steam-heated air to the drying kilns.

Towards midnight, Peel stepped out of the boiler room to cool off. The temperature has not dropped much, but he was covered in a cold sweat. He didn't feel well, and the heartburn had worsened to a burning, squeezing sensation in the center of his chest. Except for the forlorn chirruping of a cicada calling for its mate, the night was quiet. In the lull Peel noticed that the steady clickety-clack of the conveyor belt had ceased. As he rose to check the belt's mechanism, a sudden dizziness made him close his eyes and lean over. When the dizzy spell passed, he stepped into the boiler room. Spanner in hand, he climbed the narrow metal ladder to the top of the hopper where he could reach the conveyor belt and work it loose. As he bent forward, something hit him in the chest with the force of a jackhammer.

When Gladys Peel opened her eyes, the bands of sunlight slicing through the pines announced the start of a new day. Clutching the quilt to her chest, she stared at the vacant spot on the left side where her husband should have been in his accustomed place. Woodrow was a creature of habit; each night he returned from his shift at exactly 2:45 a.m., took off his boots by the kitchen door, dropped his soiled work clothes in the hamper, then tiptoed into the bedroom and slipped into bed without disturbing her.

Slipping on her robe, Gladys walked out onto the front porch and called for him, setting the neighborhood dogs barking. At six o'clock she had consumed more coffee than was good for her, and Woodrow was still missing. With shaking hands, she called Mr. Carver, the plant manager, and left a message on his answering machine. Then she called her nephew Jesse, who confirmed that her husband had given him the sandwiches she had sent. Next, she called Leroy, a friend who worked the night shift with Peel, who said he did not notice Woodrow checking out. Throwing on her clothes she grabbed her purse and headed for the sawmill.

When she arrived, the security guard at the entrance gazed at her in surprise, shaking his head in disbelief at Peel's disappearance, because he was known for his punctuality. Mounting the wooden stairs to Mr. Carver's glass enclosed-office, perched like an observation tower above the plant, she knocked on the door, with the letters SUPERINTENDENT CARVER proclaiming themselves in brass, stepped inside and blurted out that Peel had not come home. Carver reassured her that his men were looking for Peel, and if he was at the mill, they'd find him. Mr. Carver advised her to call around to friends, the church, or any place her husband might have gone.

On her way home, Gladys passed the shops on Main Street in a daze, hurried through the railroad underpass, and descended the hill leading to her neighborhood where oak trees dwarf wood frame cottages. Back in her kitchen, she started to make calls when the phone rang. Lifting the receiver to her ear, she listened, and then crumpled to her knees.

At the entrance to the sawmill, red lights pulsed into the back of Gladys's eyes. She pushed past men gathered in a tight knot around a stretcher covered in a white sheet. Her arthritic fingers reached forward to pull the sheet away. As if from a great distance, her eyes recorded what she saw. Peel lay on the stretcher gripped by rigor mortis. His faded denim overalls still fit his body as comfortably in death as in life, his worn boots were still laced securely, but his straw hat was gone. Peel's face, so animated in life, bore the mournful vacancy of death, his mouth had fallen open, and his cold eyes were turned upwards. There was no blood, but his cadaver was coated in sawdust that stuck to his hair and skin, and clogged his mouth and nose. When the hearse carrying Peel's body to the funeral home disappeared around a bend, Mr. Carver ordered everyone back to work. Back in his office, he had considered the possible consequences of Peel's death while at work. Savvy enough to smell trouble brewing, he called the company lawyer, Raymond Undershade.

Carver told the lawyer about the seventy-two-year-old employee found dead in the sawdust hopper at the Boyse Sawmill Company that morning. The lawyer fired off a salvo of questions: how come the deceased fell into the sawdust hopper? Did he slip? Was there a safety rail? Was anyone with him at the time? How long before they found him? Did the deceased have known medical problems? Did he have any enemies? What was his standing in the community? How long had he worked for the company?

The lawyer issued a warning to Carver: even if there was no foul play, there could be a violation of Occupational Safety and Health Administration (OSHA) regulations. The company could be accused of negligence. The lawyer said hat he would arrange for an autopsy to be done by an independent pathologist before the funeral—it was the only way they could protect the company from accusations of safety violations. If there had been a violation, it would be preferable to get the facts before OHSA came down on the company, or the widow sued. Raymond Undershade concluded the conversation by repeating that he would contact the pathologist immediately, and then it would be Carver's job to get the widow to sign the permission papers for the autopsy. After some hesitation, Peel's widow agreed.

In this case, the corpse of Woodrow Peel was conveyed directly to the autopsy table fully clothed and covered in sawdust. My examination of the mouth and tongue showed them to be coated in sawdust, and sawdust coated the back of the throat. His nostrils were also filled with sawdust. After the preliminary exam, my assistant removed the deceased's clothes. Upon inspection I found no evidence of external injuries. Next, the body was opened in the usual manner. Upon entry into the chest we removed the larynx, trachea, and heart in one block. The larynx and trachea where slit open along their entire length to reveal saw dust coating the vocal cords, the trachea, and the left and right bronchi. These findings suggested that Peel was still breathing when he fell into the hopper, and subsequently chocked.

After dissecting the heart in the normal manner, I opened the arteries from their origin at the aorta and discovered a clot in the left coronary artery, which supplies most of the blood to the left ventricle. All this evidence showed that Peel had collapsed as a result of a heart attack, fallen into the hopper while still breathing, inhaled the sawdust and choked to death.

When my autopsy report was delivered, Mr. Carver read every word as if his life depended on it. The summary stated:

> The Immediate cause of death is cardiac arrest as a result of a thrombotic occlusion of the left main coronary artery and resulting in acute myocardial infarction. There is evidence of sawdust inhalation secondary to the cardiac failure. This event is post cardiac and terminal.

The mention of sawdust inhalation made him uneasy. When he called, I explained that death from a thrombotic occlusion of the left coronary artery, resulting in acute myocardial infarction, meant that the blood supply to the heart muscle was blocked causing the heart muscle to die because of lack of oxygen.

"So he had a blocked artery that caused a heart attack?" Mr. Carver asked.

"That's correct. My report goes on to say that there is 'evidence of sawdust inhalation secondary to the cardiac failure, and that this event was post cardiac and terminal.' This indicates that the deceased was still breathing at the time he fell into the sawdust."

"So he had a heart attack, and that caused him to fall into the hopper?"

"The heart attack probably caused the deceased to lose consciousness and to tumble in."

Mr. Carver said, somewhat defensively, that Mr. Peel liked to fix things, that no one ordered him to climb up that ladder, that he could have called the maintenance crew, and that Boyse was proud of its safety record.

I continued, "The autopsy showed long standing lung damage from smoking, and an enlarged prostate gland, not uncommon in elderly males. However, these findings were not the cause of his death; smoking did not kill him, nor did the condition of his prostate gland."

The superintendent thanked me, evidently relieved that his employee died of a heart attack.

Afterwards, I mulled over why Peel had ignored the symptoms of heart attack. If I were to venture an educated guess, I would say that Peel did not recognize the clinical warning signs because he did not recognize what they were. To receive help on time, one should take the following symptoms seriously: a feeling of burning, discomfort or heaviness in the chest that gradually elevates; discomfort in one or both arms, the back, neck, jaw or stomach; and shortness of breath with or without chest pain. Other signs may include breaking out in a cold sweat, nausea or lightheadedness. However, there are instances of silent heart attacks, therefore it is important to have an annual check-up and periodic heart evaluations, especially as one ages.

6

Death by Motorcycle?

Bruce Lee Kung was significantly overweight at the time of his demise, yet obesity was not a direct cause of his death; it was a predictive factor, which increased his risk of developing serious complications. Piecing together Bruce's life story, I saw how it illustrated the law of unintended consequences, or outcomes different from the results intended; in hindsight, however, one could made a reasonable prediction that Lee Kung's actions in life had a high probability of leading to adverse, even fatal, results.

Named in honor of the famous martial arts movie star, Bruce descended from a long-line of karate masters. His father,

Akiro Lee Kung, a sixth degree black belt, ran a karate school. His sons, Bruce and George, were trained in the martial arts from an early age. While George excelled, Bruce, the oldest, lacked the agility or the temperament to be successful at martial arts. Still, his parents insisted that Bruce could master karate if he had the discipline to do so. There was a payoff to being a member of the Lee Kung family; most kids respected Bruce because of his folks' prowess.

On Bruce's sixteenth birthday, he got up the nerve to take the exam for the black belt; he needed to prove himself because by this time his younger brother had already achieved a black belt. As the day of the test approached, he grew more and more apprehensive.

At the start of the exam routine, Bruce performed the moves smoothly and adequately. Then towards the end, when the judge instructed them to do four repetitions of a set combination, Bruce ended up skipping the third repetition to keep up with the others. To make up for his mistake, he wanted to impress the instructor by trying more difficult sparring defenses; as a result, Bruce's moves became so aggressive that the referee gave the signal for excessive contact. Despite the warning, Bruce's next move was equally aggressive. In response, his opponent attempted to block Bruce's attack by demonstrating a strike meant to hit the opponent underneath his chin with the back of the wrist. Bruce failed to protect himself, and the blow landed squarely on his nose causing him to fall and hit his skull on the floor.

When Bruce woke in a hospital several hours later, he could not recall what had happened. The accident impaired his short-term memory, and permanently damaged his peripheral vision on the right side, and left him feeling like a miserable failure. Bruce's parents encouraged him to continue karate but he refused to do so. To their dismay, he retreated to violent video games, watched television for hours, and gained a great deal of weight, a problem that would dog him for the rest of his life. His father bought him a motorcycle just to get him out of the house, and was delighted when Bruce took to motorcycling. When the boy's mother voiced her concerns about the dangers of riding a motorcycle, especially with impaired vision, his father retorted that it provided the thrill and prowess his son had failed to find in karate.

Father and son often rode into the desert at daredevil speed. Entranced by intense desert light accentuating colors and shapes and bathing the amazing variety of cacti in a golden halo, Bruce developed an interest in the propagation of cacti. Although prohibited by law, he dug out tiny cacti with his penknife to plant behind the house. He rationalized that although he poached cactus on the U.S. Endangered Species List, he only took the youngest plants, replanting their offspring back in their native habitat.

After graduating from high school, Bruce found a job in sales at the local motorcycle dealership. There he met Mary Still Water, his future wife, who worked in town at a local art gallery that catered to tourists and produced traditional Native American baskets of excellent quality. When Bruce took her for a test run on the motorcycle, her whoops of delight as they flew through the countryside at breakneck speed spurred him on. After they married, Bruce continued to propagate cacti, telling his wife that it gave him a sense of peace with the natural world.

One spring day while riding in the desert, Bruce hit a boulder, flew over the handlebars, and landed headfirst. Discovered by a ranger hours later, he was rushed to the nearest trauma center. He sustained a skull fracture and several rib fractures. After three days in the hospital, Bruce was released.

He ached all over, and spent most of the time on the couch staring at the TV. After mopping around for days, he decided to work in his cactus garden. Mary wondered if it was wise for him to toil in the heat, but thought gardening would help him. When she next glanced out the window, she saw Bruce sprawled on the ground. She raced outside and knelt beside him. With a strange, lopsided smile contorting his face, he mumbled that he would be okay. Alarmed, she frantically called 911, but he passed away before the paramedics arrived.

Mrs. Lee Kung could not understand what had caused her husband's sudden demise. In his late thirties, he seemed too young for a heart attack. She wondered if his death had been caused by the injuries sustained in the motorcycle accident. Her sister, Lydia Pesata, a nurse who worked at the hospital in town, said that an autopsy would provide the answers she was seeking. After much soul-searching about violating her clan's traditions, Mrs. Lee Kung gave authorization for the autopsy.

Upon examining the organs, I observed that the heart was enlarged due to hypertrophy, or thickening of the left ventricular muscle wall. In the pulmonary artery I found a large clot of blood blocking the right pulmonary artery. Later in the procedure, when I opened the deep veins in the lower abdomen, pelvis and thighs, I discovered that they were filled with blood clots.

When I had removed my surgical scrubs, and cleaned up and was about to leave, Duane handed me large paper sack of unshelled pecans from the mature pecan tree in his backyard, something he did every year at the end of fall. In all the years I had known him, he said little about himself, his personal interests, or his family, only occasionally letting drop something about his church, or his grandchildren.

When she received my findings, with the aid of a medical dictionary borrowed from her sister, Mrs. Lee Kung tried to make sense of what had caused her husband's sudden death. My findings were:

> The immediate cause of death is a right pulmonary embolus totally occluding the right pulmonary artery and its major branches. There is also acute pulmonary edema and recent fracture of the right anterior 2nd and 3rd ribs. Associated pathologic findings include severe left and right coronary atherosclerotic disease, massive left ventricular hypertrophy and obesity with diffuse grade III fatty metamorphosis of the liver. In addition there is a left subdural hemorrhage and evidence of old injury to the right cerebral cortex and occipital cortex.

At a meeting in my office with Mrs. Lee Kung, I explained that an embolus usually originates from blood clots that develop in the deep veins of the legs, thighs or pelvis. Her husband's embolus originated from a deep vein thrombosis, or blood clot, in the left and right iliac veins. When the clot broke loose it traveled through the right side of the heart where it obstructed blood flow to the lungs and resulted in death.

The widow wanted to know if the doctors could have done anything to prevent the blood clot from shooting into his lungs. I told her that if his doctors had found the clot, they would have prescribed blood-thinning medicine, and advised him to keep his leg elevated when possible, wear tight-fitting elastic stockings, and to take walks. Unfortunately, the blood clot had not been detected during her husband's stay in the hospital. She questioned why the doctor hadn't found the embolus, and why they let him out of the hospital if he was in danger. I responded that at the time of her husband's discharge, he probably did not appear to need further treatment, and that in all probability there were no clinical signs to suggest deep vein thrombosis, such as swelling or discoloration of the legs, ankles or feet.

She then wanted to know about the coronary atherosclerotic disease and obesity, and I explained that my findings revealed that he was overweight with preexisting fatty plates in the walls of his coronary arteries. However, the blood clot to his lungs—not these other pathological conditions—had caused his death. When she left my office, I regretted that my report had not entirely provided Mrs. Lee Kung with the peace of mind she had hoped for. A few days later, I received a letter from an insurance company:

> We are presently evaluating a benefit request on the life of Bruce Lee Kung. Your assistance is needed in providing us with some additional information before we can continue this evaluation. We have been furnished a copy of your

Autopsy Report. In your opinion, was the manner of death in this case natural or accidental? If you feel that the manner of death was accidental, please advise if the injuries from the accident alone were sufficient to produce death. We are sending an Authorization for the release of this information.

In response, I dictated a letter into a tape recorder for my secretary to type up:

The immediate cause of death was a pulmonary embolus to the right lung with total occlusion of the artery supplying the lung. The origin of the embolus is from a deep vein thrombosis involving the left and right iliac veins. Thrombosis of deep veins is usually related to severe illness, bed rest and/or accidental trauma with subsequent hospitalization with immobilization. The pulmonary embolus is a common complication occurring in these situations. While the injuries from the accident did not cause his death, I think the accident led to the complication of deep vein thrombosis and subsequent death. If you need to discuss this with me any further I would be happy to talk with you.

As a courtesy, I asked that my secretary send a copy to Mrs. Lee Kung. Afterwards she called to tell me that she was grateful to receive double indemnity, money needed to help the children through college. Still she had regrets. If she had insisted that her husband go on a diet to lose the excess weight and quit riding his motorcycle, perhaps he might have been alive today.

I did not feel it appropriate to tell her that my report established the medical cause of death but not the psychological roots—her husband's need to prove his prowess by riding his motorcycle, a high-risk activity.

Heart disease and stroke are the leading causes of death and disability for people in the U.S. Studies reveal that overweight people are twice as likely to have high blood pressure, a major risk factor for heart disease. Very high blood levels of cholesterol can also lead to heart disease and are often linked to being overweight. Obesity contributes to angina (chest pain caused by decreased oxygen to the heart) and sudden death from heart disease or stroke without warning symptoms. On the positive side, losing a small amount of weight, around 10%, can reduce your risk of developing heart disease or a stroke.

7

Guilt by Transference

Occasionally I have been contracted to do an autopsy by a member of the family who believes that their loved one died as a result of the caregiver's negligence, or even abuse. The Merrill family's case demonstrates how deep-seated resentment between relatives can impede the acceptance of the cause of death, conclusive findings to the contrary.

Cindy Merrill placed the pills—a blood-thinner, digoxin for congestive heart failure, and a diuretic—on her mother's bedside table next to the water tumbler, at the same time making a mental note to administer the other medications after dinner—Naprosyn for arthritis, Citracal for bone loss, and Lescol for high cholesterol.

Three years ago, her mother had begun complaining of shortness of breath when she climbed the stairs, dizziness when got up from a chair, and that her feet swelled so that she had difficulty putting on her shoes. She could not lie flat without feeling that she would suffocate, finding relief only when she propped herself up on several pillows. Doctors had diagnosed congestive heart failure, and put her on medication to alleviate her symptoms. With Mother's health deteriorating rapidly, Ms. Merrill had moved back home to take care of her.

Her brother, Giles Merrill, living in Los Angeles, came to visit infrequently, and when he did he found fault with the way she took care of their mother. Although she and Giles had been close as children, as teenagers, things had gone awry between them. When Giles had finally admitted to being gay, she had reacted with hurt, anger, and disgust, as a result he had never "come out" to their mother.

On his last visit home, Giles found his mother pale and gasping for breath. Alarmed, he told his sister to call an ambulance, but she had reassured him that their mother would be fine after she took her pills. After a while, the sick woman had fallen into a deep sleep with her mouth open and snoring loudly.

Concerned that his sister was overdosing their mother, before Giles left for home he took inventory of the medications in the bathroom cabinet. When he returned to the west coast, he consulted his doctor to find out more about the drugs his mother was taking. Despite the doctor's assurance that these were appropriate mediations, Mr. Merrill could not shake the feeling that his sister was administering drugs and painkillers far too liberally.

When his sister called, a few weeks later, to tell her brother that their mother had passed away, he immediately boarded the plane, and then took a taxi straight to the funeral home. The home sat on a neat green rectangle of lawn devoid of trees. Built of limestone and red brick, with lead paned windows, and a blue slate roof, Merrill noted with approval that it was the most distinctive building in a monotonous cityscape of generic office towers.

He thought that his mother looked strangely peaceful, although her eyes were sunken and there were purple bruises on her hands. Her passing had left unfinished business and bitter regrets because he had broken his promise to reveal everything to his mother—when the time was right. His guilt turned to anger when he read his mother's will, revised just two days prior to her death:

To my son Giles, I leave only the family Bible so that he may read it daily and see the error of his ways. I bear no malice toward him, but I cannot forgive his deceiving me all these years, and I cannot condone that he has chosen to live in sin.

The one thing he had always counted on was Mother's adoration. To him it seemed obvious that his sister had revealed the secret of his homosexuality; why else would Mother have cut him out of her will so shortly before her death? Convinced that his sister Cindy was behind his mother's change of heart, and that she was also instrumental in hastening her death, he consulted a lawyer. The lawyer advised him that he would need proof to support such serious allegations of misconduct; and that an autopsy might help to provide evidence of his claim of a drug overdose. Since Giles Merrill did not have the power of attorney for his mother, he would need a court order to override his sister's objection to an autopsy. Two days later, the lawyer called Giles to let him know that he has obtained an enabling court order to perform an unlimited autopsy.

In a long conversation with me, Mr. Merrill expressed his concerns and suspicions about his sister's lax management of their late mother. I cautioned him that while I could provide a definite cause of death, my findings might or might not "prove" that his sister had done anything wrong. Still, Giles signed the authorization to proceed with the autopsy, including a toxicologic analysis.

On autopsy we found that the right coronary artery half a centimeter from its origin, was thick, hard and calcified. Cutting into the artery revealed that a 60% narrowing of the lumen, or opening, by fatty, calcified deposits in the wall. Furthermore a blood clot had blocked the narrowed opening of the artery, thus effectively cutting of the blood supply to the heart muscle. The remaining organs showed no major pathology.

The toxicological analysis, conducted by a forensic laboratory, delayed my report by three weeks.

Final Anatomical Diagnoses:
Arteriosclerotic cardiovascular disease with:
    A. Coronary arteriosclerosis, severe with thrombosis of the proximal portion of right coronary artery.
    B. Myocardial fibrosis, diffuse, moderate.
    C. Atherosclerosis, aorta, moderate.
    D. Cerebral arteriosclerosis, mild.
    E. Arterionephrosclerosis, mild.
    F. Clinical history of congestive heart failure.
        II. Pulmonary congestion, marked.
        III. Cholelithiasis

IV. Postmortem toxicologic analyses:

A. Blood opiate level of 0.3 mg/L (within therapeutic range).

B. Toxicology screens negative for elevated drug levels.

Cause of Death: Acute myocardial infarction due to thrombosis of the right coronary artery.

Case Summary: Postmortem examination to include a complete autopsy, microscopic examination of tissue sections and toxicologic analysis was performed. Autopsy revealed a severe degree of coronary arteriosclerosis with evidence of recent thrombosis of the proximal portion of the right coronary artery. This finding provides adequate explanation for the death of this individual. No evidence of trauma was detected. Nor were any findings suggestive of abuse or neglect found. Toxicological analyses revealed the presence of opiates at a level within the therapeutic range. Elevated levels of prescribed medications were not detected.

Mr. Merrill needed to confirm whether or not my report provided any verification that his sister was guilty of any wrongdoing. When he called from his cell phone in Los Angeles, I explained that his mother had a heart condition caused by narrowing of the major arteries supplying the heart with oxygen and nutrition. Damage to the heart muscles indicated that this was a long-standing problem. These findings caused congestive heart failure, for which she had received appropriate medications. The thrombosis, or blood clots, in the coronary artery were a recent development and that is what caused her death. The deceased also suffered from the formation of gallstones in her gall bladder, a condition called cholelithiasis. This resulted in abdominal pain, especially after eating fatty foods, but was not a cause of death. The postmortem blood analysis indicated that there were no abnormal substances in her blood. Some opiates, drugs in the family of morphine and its derivatives, were found at a very low level, which could not have endangered her life. No evidence of trauma, bedsores, or other signs of abuse or neglect could be detected. The cause of death was natural and related to the vascular disease present in her heart.

Mr. Merrill responded that despite these results, he still believed that his sister had something to do with his mother's death, either by withholding her medication or more likely, giving her an overdose. He called me several times over the next few months to go over the autopsy report in the hope that we would find something that would expose his sister's culpability.

In the meantime, Ms. Merrill called to thank me for proving that she did nothing wrong. She confessed that she had been resentful of her mother's overwhelming pride and unquestioning love for her Giles, despite the fact that he hardly ever came to visit, and that in a moment of anger she had blurted out the truth about her brother. She believed, however, that if her brother had found the courage to tell their mother that he was gay years ago, the recent shock of hearing about it from her would not have been so great. I replied that nothing in the autopsy report revealed that their mother died of shock.

Despite the conclusive findings at autopsy, Giles Merrill could not put his mother's death to rest. He kept on calling, still hoping to find some evidence of his sister's misdemeanors. Instead of being grateful to the immediate caregiver, relatives like Giles Merrill often try to alleviate their consciences by replacing critical hands-on care with over-zealous criticism, accusing the caretaker of negligence that has no real foundation. Perhaps the psychological mechanism at work in Gile's case was an attempt to expiate his own guilt by transferring it onto his sister.

8

Denial

Even when the clinical diagnosis of the illness that resulted in the death of a loved one is straightforward and unambiguous, I have been called upon to do an autopsy because the bereaved is convinced that the physician has been in error. Mrs. Marie Duke contracted me to do an autopsy because she sought proof that her diagnosis of her husband's illness, not the doctor's, was correct—despite all evidence to the contrary. Whatever Mrs. Duke believed, my role is an impartial one: to provide only the facts uncovered during postmortem examination.

I could tell that Mrs. Duke was having difficulty focusing on what I was saying. It was as if her mind were running backwards, like a clock losing time. While I provided her with and explanation of my findings, she kept on repeating that too many strange things happened to her husband, James Duke while in the hospital, and that the staff gave him too many drugs.

Without waiting for me to reply, she went on to tell me about her late husband's difficulty in swallowing food; that before he became so ill she would bring him his favorite foods; that he had a very good appetite up to the time that the hospital people put in a stomach peg, which caused all the problems. Mrs. Duke then digressed to relate that Mr. Duke worked as a backhoe operator for twenty years until his best buddy was killed in a freak accident. After that he found a safer job with Killingsworth Pest Control. Mr. Duke was on the job for only two years when he came down with pneumonia. Dr. Snider, the physician who first treated him, said he needed to have a chest X-ray every six months to make sure his lungs were clear. On the first X-ray they found a spot in the right upper lung, but she and her husband had not thought it was serious. Mrs. Duke rambled on about the staff at the small regional hospital, just twenty minutes from their home, who had been so caring when her husband first became ill. They had brought him soda whenever he asked for it.

When they transferred Mr. Duke to the city hospital two hours away because he was getting worse, the staff there had been unfriendly, providing him with little personal attention. They subjected her James to strange procedures and gave him too much morphine. She paused momentarily for breath, before adding that her husband had not been an old man, only 45, and then continued her litany about the problems caused by radiation, chemotherapy, and the surgery. She wanted to know why her husband kept on getting worse after the surgery, even when the surgeon told her that he had cut out the cancer. I had gone on to explain that cancer is an uncontrolled growth of cells. I described what I had observed at autopsy:

My examination of the chest revealed that the lungs were hyper inflated, or filled with air, so that air- filled sacs with the general appearance of soap bubbles were visible; normal lungs are spongy and pink without observable air sacs. The right lung had almost entirely been replaced by a large, hard, gray-white tumor mass, similar to the cut surface of a potato. This tumor tissue had grown around the esophagus and trachea. The tumor had spread out of the lungs onto the chest wall, and the surface of the vertebral column, then spread out of the chest to infiltrate the brachial plexus, or branch of nerve fibers running from the spine at the level of the chest and neck. The growth expanded and destroyed that organ and its function, and had spread into other adjoining organs through the blood stream.

In response to this lengthy explanation, Mrs. Duke reiterated that too many bad things were done to her husband in the hospital and that they gave him too many drugs.

I restated that that the autopsy confirmed that her husband died of lung cancer, not because of mismanagement or a drug overdose. I reread my final diagnosis:

> There is an advanced and extensive squamous cell carcinoma of the right upper lung lobe growing by contiguous extension into the right pleura and the mediastinum, the central organs of the chest, and the neck, and the organs surrounding the major structures of the neck. The autopsy showed that the cancer had spread to the neck and its structures.

She responded that after the surgery her husband was short of breath; then he lost his voice and he could not swallow food. And in the end he started to go paralyzed. Since all these problems happened right after the surgery, she believed that the surgery had caused them. What's more, she informed me, when they sent her James to the city hospital he got pneumonia right after they put him on a morphine pump, and then the morphine suffocated him.

I replied that morphine was administered to alleviate his pain. If she took the time to read over the autopsy report, she would see that the immediate cause of death was acute pulmonary edema and left lower lobe bronchopneumonia. That was why her husband could not breathe. I attempted to explain, yet again, that that the growth in Mr. Duke's neck had caused his difficulty in swallowing. In addition, the autopsy showed involvement of the right brachial plexus, or network of nerves formed by the lower four cervical nerves, and a focus of metastasis to the meninges, or membranes, of the spinal cord in the region T1 to T4, which caused Mr. Duke's paralysis.

Ignoring what I had told her, she countered that just before James died, the doctors said he was having cardiac problems, however, her husband never suffered from heart problems.

Her illogical leaps of thought seemed impossible to dispel. Evidently, Mrs. Duke's lack of knowledge of basic anatomy and physiology made it difficult for her to grasp the patho-physiology of cancer. Despite my explanations, despite the autopsy report showing conclusively that Mr. Duke's symptoms were caused by the spread of cancer originating in the lungs, she continued to deny it, insisting that her husband died of an overdose of morphine.

I reminded her that in our first telephone interview she had expressed concern about morphine; as a result Mr. Duke's body fluids had been tested specifically for morphine and related drugs. The test results had shown no opiates in the deceased's blood.

She retorted that when they sent her husband to ICU, they put him on a different respirator because the one they had him on broke down and maybe that's what killed him.

Realizing that it was futile to continue the conversation, I asked Mrs. Duke send me a list of questions to which I would reply in writing. When I received the questions, I answered as follows:

1) What was the morphine level in my late husband's system? Was that level in excess of what would be normal or expected based on the fact that he was being given morphine for pain management prior to his death? Answer: Toxicologic analysis detected no morphine in the blood.

2. What other drugs or medications were present in my late husband's system and in what concentrations?
Answer: The only other drug we found present was diazepam (Valium) with a 0.08 level and nordiazepam with a level of 0.12.

Both of these levels are within acceptable therapeutic range and could not have caused his death.

3. What was the oxygen level in my late husband's system?
Answer: The oxygen level was "O" (zero) and this is what you would expect in a person who is deceased. This type of testing is not appropriate at an autopsy.

4. Were you able to determine what caused my late husband's paralysis?
Answer: Yes, we were able to determine the cause of paralysis. The cause was the growth of the tumor in and around the major nerves that supply the right arm.

5. Were you able to determine the cause or origin of the perforation or puncture wound in Mr. Duke's trachea. If so, what was the cause?
Answer: Yes, we were able to determine the cause of the puncture in the trachea. The cause here is the growth and the invasion of this organ by the malignancy or tumor.

6. Do you have the laboratory results from the tests performed on the fluids drawn from James' eye and kidneys prior to the autopsy? If so, what did the results show?
Answer: We have the results on the urine: which showed no Temazepam and Oxazepam in his blood (see enclosed copy of laboratory report from the National Medical Services). The fluid from the eyes was not tested, as there was no indication for this.

I sincerely hope that I have given you all the answers that you desire and this will help further clarify the original autopsy report.

I doubted that clarification in writing would change Mrs. Duke's mind. She seemed to feel the need to pin the blame on someone. Unfortunately, my report would not bring her peace of mind because there was no one to blame. Mrs. Duke chose to deny that a lifetime of smoking ruined her husband's health and that smoking is linked to cancer. The doctors had warned him to stop smoking, and he had cut back from three packs to one a day, but couldn't break the habit. He had a smoker's cough that was so familiar to her that it had registered no more than the sound of the appliances running in the house. She refused to admit that they should have gone for X-rays as the doctor asked them to do.

In fact, cigarette smoking is the cause of most cases of fatal lung cancer—close to 90% in men, and 80% in women. There are several other forms of cancer attributed to smoking as well, including cancer of the oral cavity, pharynx, larynx, esophagus, bladder, stomach, cervix, kidney and pancreas, and acute myeloid leukemia. Exposure to secondhand smoke significantly increases the risk of lung cancer and heart disease in nonsmokers, as well as several respiratory illnesses in young children. The U.S. Environmental Protection Agency (EPA), the National Institute of Environmental Health Science's National Toxicology Program, and the World Health Organization's International Agency for Research on Cancer (IARC) have all classified secondhand smoke as a known human carcinogen.

9

Double Indemnity

Tim Chalker's fall while picking apples in his orchard was not the cause of his death: he died of natural causes, or a naturally occurring disease process. Nevertheless, his beneficiaries tried to convince me to alter my autopsy report to prove that the accident killed him. Reconstructing the events leading up to Chalker's demise, I was struck by how guilt and greed can often distort the ability to think logically.

Chalker's last day on Earth began on a mellow autumn day, in the village of Mossville, as dense fog rose slowly from the river, curling beneath the old-iron bridge where the water runs slow and deep and tiny organisms feed on skeins of algae coiling and uncoiling to the willful tug of hidden currents. As the dawn spread across the horizon, the fog drifted lazily over the railroad to a cottage on the edge of the town.

Inside the cottage, Chalker opened the blinds and saw, in the dissipating fog, the ripe apples in his orchard begging to be harvested. Turning to Rebecca, his wife, he remarked that he needed to pick the apples before they fell from the tree. Rebecca said that she would call their son Howard to come over and do the picking, as the doctor had instructed Tim to avoid strenuous exercise or a blow to the chest.

He didn't argue with his wife. Since his first surgery ten years ago to replace a bad heart valve, she had become overly protective of him. Two years after the replacement, he experienced chest pains that shot down into his left arm and neck, and had to be rushed to the hospital. The doctor said he had a major heart attack, and that the rapid emergency response saved his life. With expensive medications, Mr. Chalker had enjoyed another eight years of reasonably good health—until just six months ago when he had needed open-heart surgery to replace the old artificial valve.

After breakfast that fatal day, Mr. Chalker had gone for his morning walk, and his wife had left for the church for her quilting bee. When Chalker returned from his walk, despite his wife's objections, he decided to pick apples. Propping the ladder against the tree, he mounted the rungs, with a canvas bucket crooked in one arm, then climbed up to a branch about seven feet from the ground. As the sun rose high and hot in the sky, he picked steadily—until, without warning, intense pain seared his chest and shot down his left arm. Gasping for breath, he lost his grip and tumbled to the ground.

When Mrs. Chalker pulled into the driveway, the loud, insistent barking of their golden retriever from the orchard sent her running across the yard to find Tim sprawled unconscious on the ground with the ladder toppled over him. When the paramedics arrived she pleaded with them to take her husband to the big city hospital an hour away, where he had previously undergone heart surgery. Instead, they rushed him to the nearby county hospital's emergency room, where he was declared dead on arrival. Later, when her son, Howard, showed her the death certificate stating that Tim Chalker had died of a heart attack, his mother refused to believe it. She felt sure that her husband had damaged his valve in the accident, and that the doctors should have performed emergency surgery to repair the valve.

Days after the funeral, Howard Chalker filed a claim against his father's life insurance policy. When he read the double indemnity clause—a provision in the life-insurance policy whereby the company agrees to pay twice the face of the contract in case of accidental death—he realized that they would need proof that his father's death was accidental. When he relayed this information to his mother, he could see the gleam of vindication in her eyes.

A few weeks later, Howard received a call from Red Sklar, their insurance agent, forewarning him that they would be receiving a letter from the insurance company denying their claim for double indemnity. Howard challenged the denial, reminding Sklar that in his claim he had documented that his father had fallen off the ladder while picking apples, and in the fall his artificial heart valve had jarred loose. The agent replied that Mr. Chalker had a long history of heart problems, and that he had talked to Tim's heart surgeon who explained that once the incision heals and the valve becomes tightly seated, it's extremely unlikely to pop out like a cork—even in a fall. The insurance company, Sklar said, had to base its decision on the medical records and the death certificate, not on anecdotal accounts of what might have happened. The Chalker's insurance agents then advised Howard that an autopsy would be the only way to get proof that the valve was detached or damaged when Mr. Chalker fell from the tree. However, Sklar warned Howard that an autopsy would be costly, and that he would need to convince his boss, Sam Hempstead, that it would be worth the expense for the company to pay for exhumation, autopsy and reburial in order to avoid a lawsuit that could end up in court. In Sklar's opinion a jury might very settle in favor of a poor widow of good character, like Mrs. Chalker. On the other hand, Tim Chalker's history of heart disease together with the hospital records indicating that he died of a heart attack could go against them.

A month later, to the insurance agent's relief, he received a memo from his boss Mr. Hempstead, allocating the money for the exhumation, autopsy, and reburial. He immediately called the Chalkers' with the good news that insurance company would retain an independent pathologist to do the autopsy, one who has no connection to the hospital, the doctors or the insurance company.

When the insurance agent called to provide me with information concerning Tim Chalker, I felt that a partial autopsy [only] to examine the deceased's chest would be necessary, as the focus of my investigation was to discover whether the artificial heart valve had been displaced.

On examination I found the heart to be enlarged, and that the normal pericardial cavity had been replaced by fibrous tissue, a condition resulting from heart surgery. The aortic valve had been replaced by an artificial valve, which was in proper position and functional. The coronary arteries were brittle and narrow, with a pinpoint sized, hardly visible lumen, or opening, which is normally about a half inch in diameter. The narrowing had severely impaired the blood supply to the heart.

When my final report arrived in the mail, Mr. Hempstead read it, paying particular attention to my conclusions. When the necessary paperwork had been completed, Mrs. Chalker received a check for the full amount of the life insurance policy, but her claim for double indemnity was denied. As a result, the widow accused the insurance company and the pathologist of conspiring against her, and demanded a copy of the autopsy report. After reading the report, she still refused to accept my findings, saying that she needed to talk me personally. At her request, I met with the Chalkers' in my office to go over my findings.

I explained that, "The immediate cause of death was acute myocardial infarction imposed on an already extensively damaged left ventricle. That means that the heart muscle died, and therefore was unable to function. The left ventricle was hypertrophied secondary to hypertension. This means that the muscles of Mr. Chalker's heart chamber were enlarged—that is how the heart responds to high blood pressure."

I paused for questions before continuing, "Further complicating the heart pathology was the advanced emphysema with secondary cor pulmonale. This means there are air pockets in the lung tissue, showing that the lungs have been damaged. This type of lung disease puts an extra strain on the heart and the chambers of the heart enlarge as a result."

Mrs. Chalker responded that her husband seemed fine on the day he died.

I went on to put in plain words that I found extensive coronary artery atherosclerosis with calcification and markedly reduced coronary artery blood flow, indicating that the vessels supplying the heart muscles with blood became narrow and brittle and were therefore unable to supply sufficient blood to the heart muscles.

Both mother and son look stunned when I told them that Tim Chalker's prosthetic aortic valve was properly seated and functional. This meant that the valve was in the right place, properly anchored, and was in working order.

Mrs. Chalker retorted that she still believed that the valve must have gotten loose when her husband fell off the ladder, and that she is planning to consult a lawyer. Soon after that she sent a letter to the State Medical Association and State Insurance Commissioner. The concluding paragraph read:

> I really think that the emergency room doctor and the pathologist should be investigated. I feel they should revise their reports. The pathologist said that the valve was functioning but I wonder if it broke loose in the accident.

I feel like the valve in Tim's heart was damaged and I'm not sure how the doctor determined it was good. It seems he could have found out that it might have been damaged because of the fall. Would you please advise me what you are going to do?

The case never came to trial. The state medical board and state insurance commission found the autopsy report to be in order. Mrs. Chalker had no further recourse. The case was closed, but Mrs. Chalker and her son were never able to put it to rest.

10

A Subtle Case of Neglect

Thanks to medical advances, people are enjoying longer life spans than any time in history. However, aging parents and grandparents often require daily assistance, thereby presenting a challenge to find appropriate and affordable help. My autopsy on Jim McHale highlighted the need for caregivers to receive counseling on how best to take care of an elderly parent living alone.

On the last day of February, Priscilla Sexton, older daughter of Jim McHale, stands in the sunroom enjoying the seemingly impromptu appearance of yellow daffodils poking through brown winter leaves. As she contemplates her chores for the day, she reflects that she hasn't seen her father, Jim McHale, in over three days. She dreads her visits to him. He is often in a bad mood, or rambles on about his achievements as secretary of the Detroit Building & Construction Trades Council, an office he held for 15 years. She decides to put off her visit to her father to the next day. First thing tomorrow, she vows that she will cook a pot of her father's favorite Texas chili and bring it to him.

Across town, McHale sits in his recliner, parked in front of the TV, enjoying a beer while watching the Atlanta Braves clobber the Florida Marlins. He's running low on groceries, but he's too proud to call Priscilla, his older daughter, or Mary his younger daughter, although they were the ones who insisted he move to Atlanta, away from his familiar neighborhood and the buddies he had known all his life. Now he spends most of the time resting, because his weakened legs will not carry him far.

Heaving himself from the recliner with some difficulty, he shuffles over to his old wooden desk and pulls open the bottom drawer to reveal a hoard of small round tins containing custom chewing tobacco. With trembling fingers he shoves a wad inside his left cheek and settles himself back in the recliner with a grunt. During the fifth inning, the back of his throat starts to hurt, a phlegmy cough rises in his throat, and the pain in his chest feels worse. When the coughing subsides, he is exhausted and falls into a restless sleep. Hours later McHale wakes to the crackling of static on the TV, shivering and hacking; his chest is so tight he can barely breathe. With difficulty, he staggers to the bedroom, curls up on the bed, and pulls a worn quilt over his head. Another attack of coughing seems to be tearing his lungs from his chest. The fever in him burns higher lifting his mind on the parabolic waves of time, sweeping him deeper and deeper into the past.

On the day she plans to visit her father—and four days since she has last seen him—the phone rings just as Mrs. Sexton steps out of the shower. It's Joel Smith, her father's next-door neighbor, calling to tell her that Jim McHale isn't answering the doorbell or the telephone, but he can hear the TV running.

Mrs. Sexton arrives at her father's apartment to find emergency vehicles and the police parked outside. Inside the apartment she fights the urge to throw up as a sickly smell assails her. McHale's full-clothed body is curled rigidly into a fetal position with his knees drawn up to his chin. Blood mixed with mucus has trickled down the stubble on his chin, and onto the soiled sheets.

Across the country in Seattle, Mary McHale, Mr. McHale's younger daughter, receives a call from her brother-in-law, Walker Sexton, with the news of her father's demise. She immediately books a flight to Atlanta. Eight months before, Ms. McHale had called her sister to voice her concern about their father's deteriorating health, and the poor circumstances in which he was living in Detroit. He had neglected the old house, and the neighborhood had become dangerous. At his daughters' insistence, McHale sold the house and agreed to move to Atlanta to be near his older daughter, Mrs. Sexton.

As the plane drones through the air, Ms. McHale blames herself for not monitoring her Dad's situation more closely. From what she can gather, he had been dead for at least two or three days before police broke into his apartment.

Outside baggage claim, Mary's sister, Priscilla, and her brother-in-law are waiting to drive her to the Jefferson Funeral Home, on the south side of downtown. The home sits on a green rectangle of lawn devoid of trees. Built of limestone and red brick, with lead paned windows, and a blue slate roof, it is the most distinctive building in a monotonous cityscape of office blocks.

The funeral director, wearing a dark suit and matching tie, leads Ms. McHale to the preparation room. Her father's remains lie on a gleaming stainless steel slab. Other than a coarse white sheet, no shroud shields his body from prying eyes. She shudders as the funeral director pulls down the sheet to expose the head and chest. The circumstances surrounding her father's death and her feelings of guilt fuel her grief and anger. That he should have died in such a pitiful state, without medical intervention, is painful to accept.

Turning to her older sister, the younger sister, Mary, blurts out that if Priscilla had had looked in on him more often, their father might have received medical attention, but it's too late now. Ms. McHale informs her sister that she intends to authorize an autopsy to find out what killed their father. Practiced in the art of handling his wife—now sobbing bitterly—Walker Sexton suggests that an autopsy might indeed put an end to speculation; it will confirm that his father-in-law died of an incurable disease, in which case they cannot blame themselves for the inevitable.

After listening to the events prior to Mr. McHale's death, I determine that only a partial autopsy is necessary because the organs of interest are the brain and the chest; the examination of these organs together with a good clinical history should answer the unresolved issues; and this limited procedure is also less costly.

The McHale sisters are relieved when I assure them that they can go ahead with the funeral the next day. I explain that at the culmination of the service the casket will be lowered into the grave, but will not be buried. When everyone has departed, the body will be transported back to the funeral home for the autopsy. When the autopsy is completed, the casket with Jim McHale's remains will be taken back to the cemetery for proper burial.

At postmortem, I noted the skeletal appearance of an individual who appeared not to have had sufficient nourishment for months. A large skin ulcer over the lower back and buttocks exuded greenish-yellow pus. The lungs were dark red, hard and beefy, instead of pink and spongy. When I compressed the cut surface of the lungs with my gloved fingers, small beads of yellow pus exuded from the bronchioles, or air tubes.

Their father's funeral brings no closure to the sisters, no emotional resolution to this traumatic event in their lives. They both, privately, hope that the autopsy will expunge some of the guilt they are feeling.

When my final report arrives in the mail Ms. McHale wades through the medical terminology. Postmortem Examination:

The daughter of the deceased has signed authorization for unlimited autopsy. The permit is properly witnessed. A funeral home identification tag around the left ankle identifies the body.

Then follows a detailed description of the external appearance and the internal organs. The last page is the most relevant to the McHale sisters.

Final Anatomical Diagnoses:

I. Clinical history of Multiple Sclerosis with:

A. Lobar pneumonia, upper and lower lobes of right lung.

B. Cachexia, marked.

C. Decubitus ulcers, sacrum and buttocks, multiple, large.

D. Patchy demyelinization of white matter, brainstem and cervical spinal cord, focal, mild.

E. Fecal impaction, distal colon.

Conclusion:

Cachexia and inanition with lobar pneumonia due to complications associated with Multiple Sclerosis.

When Mary McHale finishes the report she puts both hands on her head and rocks from side to side. She knows what pneumonia is, but what is cachexia, what is Multiple Sclerosis? It won't be enough to look up these words in a medical dictionary; she needs to talk directly to the pathologist who performed the autopsy.

To her relief, she reaches me on her first call so that I can proceed to clarify my findings.

"Mr. McHale's right lung was infected with bacteria that cause pneumonia. In older people, this is can be fatal if left untreated," I tell her.

"So he died of pneumonia?"

"Yes, he did. Your father was also suffering from cachexia, or severe malnutrition with marked weight loss brought on by chronic disease."

"I see. But he was always a picky eater. He even complained about my sister's good home cooking," she says.

"The malnutrition was exacerbated by chronic illness," I clarify, before continuing, "Mr. McHale also had bedsores as a result of immobility. Bedsores are dead areas of the skin, with ulceration and infection caused by lying in the same position too long."

This time an excuse doesn't come readily to mind, and Ms. McHale remains silent.

"As I said, your father died of untreated pneumonia. However, severe malnutrition, and Multiple Sclerosis were contributing factors that hastened his death."

"Multiple Sclerosis?"

I am surprised that she didn't know he suffered from this illness.

"My father was fiercely independent and a very private man. I suppose he didn't want us to know there was something wrong with him."

"Did you notice his increasing difficulty in getting around?"

"Yes, but I-I, thought it was just due to old age," she stammers.

"MS is a chronic disease of the nervous system with deterioration of the nerve fibers. He had this disease for many years," I say.

"Doctor, we did what we could for my father, but he refused help. He could be obstinate and bad-tempered."

As I put down the phone, I pity the sisters, who will live with guilt for the rest of their lives. Theirs was a subtle form of neglect that created a high-risk situation. Studies show that as the over-65 age group approaches 20% of the total US population, the pressure to meet the social and health care of the elderly will escalate. Every year an estimated 2.1 million older Americans are victims of physical, psychological, or other forms of abuse or neglect. Recent research suggests that elders who have been mistreated or neglected tend to die earlier than those who have proper care, even in the absence of chronic conditions or life-threatening disease. What can be done to alleviate this unfortunate situation? In my opinion, caregivers should be provided with supportive counseling services from health professionals and, where possible, financial assistance if needed.

11

The Homeless Rastafarian

The ravages of a homeless existence were starkly evident on the corpse of 39-year-old Victor Torres. However, while performing the postmortem, I did not speculate on what sort of person he had been while alive; the immediate task at hand was to learn what had caused his death. Later, there would be time for such conjecture:

Around ten o'clock on Friday night, the man in a black ski cap and dark glasses limped up to the emergency desk at Brixton Medical Center. The admission clerk/receptionist, Velma

Thorsby, smelled the rank odor of stale nicotine, liquor, dirty clothing and unwashed flesh before she saw him. She looked up sharply and scrutinized the man with a long, angular face, red-splotched cheeks and a purple nose, wearing a ragged duffle coat buttoned over several layers of clothing. Although Nurse Thorsby did not recall his name, she recognized him from previous visits as one of the many homeless addicts who used the hospital's emergency facilities to get shelter and assistance when they were desperate.

"I'm sick, get me a doctor," he snarled, then doubled over and threw up, as he did so his cap came off revealing an unkempt-head of hair resembling matted Rastafarian dreadlocks.

Nurse Thorsby paged Nurse Brooks, the emergency nurse on call. Nurse Brooks checked the man's vital signs, and cleaned vomit from his face and mouth to clear any obstruction. The man remained passive as he was lifted onto the gurney, but when the orderly began to strap him down he became agitated.

Nurse Thorsby watched thoughtfully as they wheeled the patient to the examination room. Working in a big city hospital she had seen more than her share of homeless substance abusers. Years of chronic drinking and drugs always exacted a heavy toll on their health, and although they were in desperate need of medical services, they rarely had health insurance. This harsh reality forced them to ignore health problems for immediate survival on the street. Unfortunately, deferring health care resulted in expensive treatment in hospital emergency rooms subsidized by taxpayers and the health insurance system.

In the examination room, Nurse Brooks stripped off the man's soiled shirt, jeans and shoes, although he resisted. She was relieved when Dr. Mulvane, the young intern, arrived. Ignoring the man's threatening glare, he asked where he was feeling pain. The patient replied that he had terrible burning pain in his stomach, and had been vomiting all day. When Dr. Mulvane palpated his abdomen, the man winced. The monitor lit up with a watery green glow, and Dr. Mulvane took a moment to look at the EKG, noting the heart rate, breathing rate, and blood pressure scrolling across it.

Nurse Thorsby came through the swinging doors and handed a blue folder to Dr. Mulvane, commenting that this patient had been seen in the emergency room previously. The intern scanned the medical charts and notes, which included the report of Cornelius Eddy, a drug counselor at the Asheville detox center. Evidently, the patient's name was Victor Torres, age 39, who had been treated at the center for his addiction to the painkiller OxyContin.

Bringing his knees to his chest, the man groaned, "Give me something to stop the pain."

Dr. Mulvane wrote a prescription for Tagamet, to alleviate Mr. Torres' discomfort. Then he ordered tests to find what was causing the patient's symptoms. In light of the patients' history of drug abuse, Dr. Mulvane considered the host of ailments he could have developed: including pancreatitis, gastritis or ulcers, malnutrition, tuberculosis or AIDS. Just to be on the safe side, the doctor asked the ER nurse to set up an IV and to attach the patient to a monitor to track his vital signs. As the nurse attempted to find a vein to cannulate, she noticed the needle marks puncturing the patient's arm. Before he left, Dr. Mulvane asked Nurse Brooks to draw blood to send to the lab for a panel of tests, and then scribbled a note to the lab tech to call him when the results were ready. Although it was hospital policy to release indigent patients such as Mr. Torres as soon as possible, the intern made the decision to admit the patient overnight, primarily because he wanted time to get him into drug treatment.

Soon after Mr. Torres had been transferred to a hospital ward, three victims of a car crash were brought into the ER, which kept the intern busy for most of the night. Just before he went off duty, the lab tech called to say that Mr. Torres' lab tests were normal. Despite his fatigue, Dr. Mulvane made a call to the drug counselor who had treated Victor Torres previously.

The counselor told him that Torres' problems had begun back in high school when he joined the Rastafarians, who used marijuana as part of their cult.

Last fall, police in Asheville found Mr. Torres stoned and bumming around for food. They took him to the state psychiatric hospital. Several months later, he showed up at an alcohol and drug abuse treatment center near Asheville declaring that he was going to die. After treatment at the Asheville center, Mr. Torres stayed clean for a few months. But he could not hold down a job and reverted to sleeping in crack houses. He bought drugs by selling drugs.

The young intern listened to what the counselor had to say, and then responded that before he had discharged Torres, he wanted to get him into treatment. The counselor recommended a shelter near the hospital. With some difficulty, Dr. Mulvane persuaded Mr. Torres to go the shelter when he was discharged. Satisfied that there was nothing more he could do for the patient, the intern told Torres to make an appointment for a check up the following week, and to stay away from alcohol and drugs. After that he prepared the discharge papers.

On exiting the hospital an hour later, Mr. Torres asked a passerby on the parking lot for a match to light a cigarette. Leary of his rough appearance, the woman shook her head and hurried on. When she heard the man retching violently, she turned and saw him crumple to the ground. She quickly alerted the nurse at the front desk. Within minutes, the Emergency Medical Team administered CPR to Mr. Torres on the parking lot. Unable to revive him, they rushed him into the ER where they continued resuscitation to no avail.

    The only identification to be found on Mr. Torres was the hospital's prescription note for Tagamet with Dr. Mulvane's signature. They hospital administrator, Marsha Mitford, was alerted to the situation. Concerned that the patient had died on the hospital parking lot just minutes after being discharged, and just hours after being admitted to the hospital, she immediately scheduled conferences with Dr. Mulvane, Nurse Thorsby, and Nurse Brooks. As Brixton was a small community hospital with no pathologist on staff, she then arranged for me to perform an autopsy. Mrs. Mitford also requested that the chief medical officer review Victor Torres' medical history and the events prior to his demise.

    Dr. Mulvane returned home from ER exhausted and ready for sleep; however, he first listened to his phone messages in case he needed to attend to something urgently. Dismayed to hear that hospital administrator needed to meet with him concerning the death of Victor Torres, he leaned against the wall, and considered the question popping in his head. Why had the patient died so suddenly? What had caused his death?

I cut open the pericardial sac surrounding the heart, and the pulmonary artery where it exits the heart. I pushed my index finger into the hole in the pulmonary artery and felt for a thromboembolus, or blood clot, which could have dislodged from a vein somewhere else in the body, and traveled through the heart to the pulmonary artery where it became trapped, causing sudden death. I found no clot within the pulmonary artery. However, the coronary arteries were hard and brittle to the touch, and severely narrowed along their entire course, reducing the size of a pinhead, and thus greatly restricting the blood flow to the heart muscle.

By the time my autopsy report arrived on her desk, Marsha Mitford, the administrator, had gathered all pertinent information on Victor Torres, but still it did not tell her why he had died on the parking lot. My report provided the missing facts she needed. She read through the five-page report, then reread the last page and the case interpretation:

> The immediate cause of death is an extensive antero-lateral and antero-septal left ventricular myocardial infarction secondary to severe coronary atherosclerosis with calcification. The heart problem is complicated by the presence of concentric left ventricular hypertrophy. The other findings are terminal, which include the acute

bilateral lower lobe pulmonary edema and the congestion of the liver and spleen.

If she had understood correctly, the autopsy confirmed what she feared: Victor Torres died of a heart attack.

Before swinging into action, Marsha Mitford, the administrator, discussed the autopsy report with Dr. Zither, chairman of the medical review committee. The chairman first took a few minutes to read the report, with particular attention to the Final Anatomic Diagnosis, then read it aloud, adding his own explanations for clarification after each point:

"Point one. 'Acute myocardial infarction, antero-lateral and antero-septal.' In lay terms this means, death of the muscles of the heart due to blockage of the arterial supply of blood.

"Point two. 'Grade IV atherosclerosis with calcification of the coronary arteries.' In other words, the main arteries that supply the heart with blood were calcified or hardened and blocked by fatty deposit.

"Point three. 'Marked concentric left ventricular hypertrophy.' The heart had enlarged and thickened probably because of high blood pressure.

"Point four. 'Acute left and right lower lobe pulmonary edema.' Fluid accumulation in the lungs which occurs when the heart stops beating—that occurs after death.

"Point five. 'Acute terminal congestion, liver and spleen.' This also occurs when the heart stops beating.

"Point six. 'Anthracosis and focal pulmonary fibrosis.' There was deposition of carbon particles and damage to the lungs probably due to smoking.

"Point seven. 'Drug addition and alcohol abuse.' That doesn't need an explanation.

"Point eight. 'Atopic dermatitis.' That's a skin inflammation which could be due to allergy or poor hygiene."

When he had finished, Dr. Zither cleared his throat and patted his bald pate before commenting to Mrs. Mitford, that excessive use of alcohol, or abuse of drugs such as cocaine, amphetamines, and certain prescription drugs are known to place stress on the heart, or damage the cells of the heart, which can result in heart failure or other heart diseases.

The administrator scheduled a meeting of the hospital's medical review committee, including chiefs of cardiology, surgery, emergency services, and the head of nursing services. In addition, she asked the hospital cardiologist to review Torres' EKG, in order to determine why Dr. Mulvane had not detected any abnormalities.

When the committee gathered a few days later, Mrs. Mitford had collected a thick dossier on Victor Torres' case. After the administrator and chief medical officer had presented a review of the case, they asked Dr. Mulvane to respond.

The intern began by reminding them that he had been so concerned about Victor Torres' history of drug abuse that he had admitted him to hospital at the risk of being chastised, since the patient had no insurance. He had called Cornelius Eddy, Mr. Torres drug counselor in Asheville, who had arranged to find a place for him at the rehabilitation center, although it was overcrowded. He went on to explain that every year, thousands like Torres go untreated because rehab centers offering inpatient treatment lack bed space and staff. In his defense, Dr. Mulvane said that he could have washed his hands of Torres the night he came into the ER. Had he done so, the patient would have died on the streets; instead he took on the added responsibility of helping Torres find shelter and treatment.

Dr. Mitford concurred that the dire needs of homeless drug addicts were not being met, however, she stated that the intern had missed the diagnosis on Mr. Torres's EKG. If he had any doubts, he should have ordered a cardiology consult. As a result, a man whose life might have been saved had died, leaving the hospital open to being sued.

Dr. Mulvane had made the easy assumption that Victor Torres' problems were related to drug abuse, especially since he was only thirty-nine with no known history of heart problems.

Later, I received a memo from the administrator informing me that I would be deposed. I never was. Nor did I learn why, as the hospital keeps such matters confidential. I presumed that in the case of a homeless drug addict like Victor Torres, it was possible that no member of his family stepped forward to file a lawsuit.

Whatever the circumstances, the case of Victor Torres shows that efforts to reduce the use of emergency departments by the homeless must not ignore the underlying risk factors prevalent among those with alcohol and drug abuse.

12

A Case of Exhaustive Mania

When an apparently healthy young individual like William Packer dies suddenly, thousands of miles away from home, it is natural for the family to suspect malfeasance. To uncover the truth about what had happened, the deceased's younger brother, Ned Packer, authorized me to perform an autopsy. He also asked that I review the American Consulate's logbook, and the autopsy report of the Japanese pathologist, done prior to my autopsy. As I compiled the results of the autopsy, and the sequence of events preceding Packer's death in Tokyo, a tragic picture emerged of his anguish in the last hours of his life.

At precisely 8:30 in the morning, Marie Seldon, assistant to the consul at the American Embassy in Tokyo, received a bizarre call from Keisatsu Hattori, at the Nakano Police Station, informing her that they had taken a mentally ill American into custody. He appeared to be disoriented and upset, and refused to answer their questions. His clothes were torn and dirty, he wore no shoes, and he carried no wallet, or ID. Evidently, the man had climbed into the back of a woman's car while she was waiting at a stoplight. When she demanded that he get out, the American became extremely agitated and refused to budge. Since Nakano Police Station was just around the corner, the woman drove there for assistance. Hattori, who spoke some English, tried to reason with the American, but in the end had to remove him from the vehicle. The American came on the phone yelling something about it being dangerous for him to go home because someone was trying to feed off his brain. He would not give Ms. Seldon his name or to say how long he had been in Japan.

Keisatsu Hattori came back on the line to advise her that they were very busy at the police station and needed someone from the embassy to pick up the American as soon as possible. Ms. Seldon replied that they could not do that. The police needed to send the man to a medical facility as he was suffering from a mental illness. Hattori said that they could not proceed without this man's ID, or the consent of his family.

Ms. Seldon told Mr. Hatori that she would talk to her superior, Consul Delaney, and get back to him shortly. To her relief, the consul concurred with her decision that the police should transport the American to the police mental health detention center, or otherwise they should release him.

"You know," the consul said, tilting back in his chair, "each year more than 2,000 American citizens are arrested abroad and over half of those arrested are held on charges of using or possessing drugs."

"Yes, I've had to deal with Americans who got into a trouble because they assumed, incorrectly, that they were immune from prosecution in a foreign country," his assistant agreed.

The consul went on, "Over the years I've seen all sorts of misunderstandings that landed Americans in jail. A woman who purchased a curio in Turkey to get rid of a street seller was arrested for smuggling antiquities. A businesswoman in Nigeria found out that her dealings had been made illegal retroactively, and then faced a death sentence." The consul went on to assure his assistant that he did not believe this American would receive any punishment. The police had not formally arrested or charged him because they hadn't found drugs on him. Perhaps the young American's predicament would serve as a wake up call to get himself into treatment.

When Ms. Seldon returned to her desk, there was a message

from Hattori urgently reiterating that the consular office send someone to pick up the American promptly. To avoid getting into an argument with the policeman, Ms. Seldon instructed the embassy operator to repeat what she had said earlier: It was the police's responsibility to deal with the American. Since the man was in their custody, they could arrest him, or let him go. She also instructed the operator to explain that when a foreign person is arrested in the United States, they deal with that person through the legal system; they do not hand him off to their embassy.

About fifteen minutes later, the operator came back on the line to say that the police had identified the man as William Packer, born July 9, 1989. He had lived in Japan on and off for about seven years. The police repeated that they could not detain him any longer and were bringing him to the embassy.

When Ms. Seldon apprised the consul of the latest turn of events and the name of the American, he immediately recalled that about two weeks earlier, Packer had arrived at the embassy barefooted, with an ugly bruise on his cheek and a bloody nose. He was incensed that Japanese authorities had refused to renew his alien registration card and ordered him to leave the country. Consul Delaney bought him lunch and a pair of shoes, and then advised him to purchase a plane ticket back to the U.S. Delaney went on to say that while he could not prevent the police from bringing the man to the embassy, the embassy would not take him into its custody. He notified the guards that they were not authorized to let William Packer in, and instructed them to call Ms. Seldon as soon the American arrived so that she could talk to Mr. Packer to find out how she could contact a friend or a colleague to come and get him.

When Ms. Seldon expressed her concern about Packer's precarious mental state, Delaney reminded her that the American Embassy and its consular services could not act as Packer's legal advisor, or pay for his legal fees, nor his medical expenses. Ms. Seldon noted all this in her logbook, as she was required to do.

Just as she was about to leave for lunch, the operator relayed a phone call from Hattori, informing her that they were taking William Packer to a hospital, but did not specify which one. Relieved that the American would be receiving medical attention without their having to intervene, Ms. Seldon then instructed the operator to find out to which hospital they had transported William Packer.

Shortly after she returned from lunch, a friend of William Packer called, identifying himself as Barry Goldsmith. Goldsmith explained that he taught English with Packer at an after school "cram school," where Japanese high school students went for supplemental lessons. He was concerned about his friend: he hadn't seen him in two days, although he had purchased a plane ticket and should have left for the States that morning. He had left his apartment unlocked with everything he owned, including money and his expired plane ticket.

As Ms. Seldon questioned Goldsmith, the unfortunate sequence of events leading to Packer's detention by the police began to emerge. About two weeks ago, the American had tried to renew his work permit but the Japanese authorities had summarily ordered him out of the country. After that he had become extremely upset and started acting irrationally. He arrived at work obviously hung over and incapable of controlling his students.

Upon questioning, Goldsmith said that he did not believe his friend took drugs, but he did drink heavily, and he had heard rumors that he was once committed to a mental hospital. Packer had told him that his father died a few years ago, his mother had Alzheimer's, and that his younger brother lived in West Virginia. Ms. Seldon asked Goldsmith to lock up Packer's apartment, promising to call as soon as she knew where the police had taken his friend. Then she made a note of the conversation in her logbook.

Later that day, Ms. Seldon received a duty call from the embassy operator informing her that William Packer was being held at the Tokyo Immigration Center. When the immigration officer put Packer on the phone, he was abusive and irrational, yelling that he didn't want to talk to her, that he needed to talk to his brother. Before she could reply, he hung up.

Ms. Seldon asked the embassy operator to contact the immigration authorities to find out what they planned to do with Packer, and to relay her message that that someone from the embassy would visit Packer during business hours, but could not guarantee hospital bills.

She was just about to contact his friend, Barry Goldsmith, when he pre-empted her call to say that William had just telephoned to say that the police were taking him to a hospital. Goldsmith couldn't make out which hospital they were taking him to as he was yelling and crying, but said he would go to see his friend as soon as knew where he was. Immediately afterwards, the embassy operator paged Ms. Seldon with a message from the police informing her that Packer was being transported to Nansung Hospital. Ms. Seldon noted the hospital's address and phone number then asked the operator to contact the hospital and inform them that someone from the American Embassy would be coming to see Mr. Packer.

Ms. Seldon felt relieved that the American would finally get the attention he so sorely needed. She glanced at her wristwatch and saw that it was 3:15 p.m. It had been a trying day. As she turned to update her logbook, she heard herself being paged over the intercom. It was Barry Goldsmith calling to tell her that he was at Nansung Hospital, but had not been allowed to see William Packer. He had spoken to the doctor who said that they had to sedate William because he was violent and extremely agitated. Mr. Goldsmith thought that they needed to get in touch with someone from William Packer's family to let them know what was going on. Ms. Seldon replied that as an embassy official she needed a PAW, or permission of waiver, before she could do so. But since Goldsmith was not a government official, he was free to contact the family as a friend. Goldsmith said that he had found William's brother's phone number in an address book, and, although he'd called several times, no one answered. The assistant told his friend to keep on trying and to let her know of any change in Packer's situation, adding that she would visit his friend as soon as possible, but that the hospital was the safest place for his friend until his behavior stabilized.

After putting down the phone, Ms. Seldon filled out the PAW form so that she could proceed to contact Packer's family. Shortly afterwards, she received a call from the duty doctor at Nunsung Hospital, informing her that William Packer's respiration and pulse were very high and that he needed to be transferred to Adventist Hospital for lab tests, as Nansung did not have a lab.

She called Consul Delany to let him know that they were transporting Packer to the Adventist Hospital. The consul advised Ms. Seldon to keep him updated. About an hour later, Policeman Hattori called with the shocking news that William Packer had died while in transit. Delaney instructed Ms. Seldon not to call the

Packer family until they could gather more information on the cause of death.

Accompanied by Yuko Keitoku, an embassy translator, Ms. Seldon left immediately for the hospital. When she arrived, Barry Goldsmith and a friend from the "cram school" were waiting for her in a state of shock. Goldsmith told Ms. Seldon that when he had last seen William at the Nansung hospital the night before, his hands and feet had been tied to the bed, but he had appeared to be sleeping peacefully. The doctor on duty explained that because William had been violent and verbally abusive, they had to restrain and tranquilize him.

With the translator's help, Ms. Seldon interviewed the ambulance attendant who had accompanied Packer to the hospital. He said that while in transit he had checked the American's vital signs and kept his oxygen mask and IV going, although Packer repeatedly attempted to yank them out. Policeman Hattori gave his assurances that his department would investigate what had happened to William Packer and send a full report to the American Embassy. He informed her that an autopsy would be mandatory, as the doctors could not determine a cause of death, and the circumstances surrounding it were unclear. Ms. Seldon received permission to accompany the police crew to Packer's apartment to retrieve documents and other valuables in order to secure them at the embassy. Before leaving the hospital, Ms. Seldon advised the authorities that the embassy would need a copy of the Japanese death certificate so that a U.S. death certificate could be issued for William Packer.

With Ms. Seldon at his heels, Police Officer Hattori opened the door to Packer's apartment and flicked on the lights. For a moment the two stood motionless, surveying the room. Clothing, plates of half-eaten food, overturned coffee mugs, torn newspapers and empty bottles were strewn everywhere. The acrid smell of scorched material mixed with the odor of stale alcohol pervaded the air. Following Hattori's raised finger, Ms. Seldon saw stacks of partially burnt paper currency heaped onto a futon.

After gathering what was needed, Ms. Seldon took a taxi back to the embassy to turn over the backpack with Packer's personal papers, and to brief the consul on what she had gleaned thus far. She was certain that William Packer's family would have many questions about the circumstances surrounding his death. Had Packer been mistreated while in police custody? Had the doctors failed to diagnose a serious illness? What had happened to him before he came to the attention of the police? Why had Japanese Immigration ordered him to return to the U.S.? She hoped that the police investigation and the autopsy would provide the answers they needed. In addition, the consul's delay in visiting William Packer until too late concerned her personally. She knew that embassy procedure clearly states that a representative from the embassy or consul should promptly visit an American citizen who has been arrested to determine their situation.

Consul Delaney was waiting for her at the embassy to debrief her. Before she left work, he requested that she compose a fact sheet with the deceased's name, date and place of birth and death, passport number, cause of death (if available), and the location of his remains. In addition, he needed the full name and address of the next of kin and their instructions regarding funeral arrangements.

A week after William Packer's sudden demise, I received a call from Ned Packer, William's younger brother. With mounting curiosity and concern, I heard his account of the unfortunate circumstances surrounding his brother's death. Understandably, Ned Packer feared that there had been misconduct by the police, the American Consul, or even the doctors. Although the Japanese authorities had performed an autopsy on his brother before flying him home for burial, the information he had received appeared to be incomplete and misleading. As a result, Ned requested that I examine his brother to establish a cause of death independent of the Japanese authorities. In addition, he asked that I review the Japanese autopsy report, which he would have translated into English. He expected that it would take several long distance calls to cut through red tape before the report and slides could be delivered to me.

In the meantime, I proceeded with the examination of William Packer's remains, which had been shipped back to the US for burial. The external exam showed sutured incisions on his body made by the autopsy and embalming procedures. There were multiple small bruises on the face, upper extremities and abdomen, and a fading bruise over the bridge of his nose. As these bruises were small and superficial, I concluded that they were caused by flailing against his restraints during delirium, and not by directed blows. I could find no broken or fractured bones. My internal examination of the soft tissue and organs—replaced after the autopsy—revealed no abnormalities or traumatic injuries.

When the slides, photos, and the autopsy report together with transcripts of the embassy logbook arrived from Japan, I reviewed them meticulously. The autopsy, performed by the medical examiner of a Japanese government institution, was thorough. It stated that the skull was intact, and there were no bone fractures or internal hemorrhages of the brain. There was no evidence of traumatic injury, asphyxiation, or poisoning. Traces of marijuana were found in the urine. Since the Japanese pathologist could find no physical or traumatic cause of death, he concluded the cause of death as "undetermined."

I forwarded all this information to the Packer family; nevertheless, they remained suspicious that the authorities had failed William Packer. I suggested that we consult Dr. Harry Grant, a forensic pathologist, at the state forensic lab. After considering all the evidence, Dr. Grant ruled out drug overdose, as only small amounts of the degradation products of marijuana were found in the urine. Psychiatric problems were difficult to confirm. William's friend reported that he had been treated for mental illness but could not verify it. The principal of the school where Packer taught stated that just two days before he died, he showed up at the school crying and unhappy about being ordered back to United States. According to the principal, Packer had received psychiatric treatment in the past, and his treatment records had been forwarded to the police. However, the Packer family claimed that they knew nothing about William having mental problems, and were offended by that assertion.

Dr. Grant and I felt that the police reports supported the hypothesis that the American was suffering from mental instability at the time of his arrest. According to police statements, William Packer was shivering and incoherent when taken into custody. The police transferred him to Nunsang Municipal Hospital because of his extremely irrational and violent behavior, where he was placed in an isolated observation room, with his arms and legs restrained, and he was injected with tranquilizers. Later that day, the attendant on duty notified the duty doctor that Packer was in severe distress. The doctor gave orders for Packer to be transferred a city hospital with lab facilities. While in transit, William Packer tried to pull off his oxygen mask and the IV needle in his arm. He was declared dead on arrival at the hospital.

After reviewing the events preceding William Packer's demise, Dr. Grant came to the conclusion that his case showed remarkable similarities to others he had investigated. All were young men who exhibited the acute onset of irrational, aggressive behavior with incoherent or meaningless speech, and paranoid delusions. Their behavior was so extreme that in all cases they needed to be restrained and the police were called. Dr. Grant concluded that William Packer succumbed to what is known in the forensic literature as acute exhaustive mania, or excited delirium.

He ruled out Neuroleptic Malignant Syndrome (NMS), another recognized cause of sudden, or unexpected death. NMS presents in a manner very similar to exhaustive mania, generally occurring in psychiatric patients who are on antipsychotic medication. Extreme physical exhaustion, dehydration, and organic brain disease may also be predisposing factors. The symptoms include hyperthermia, or elevated body temperature, fluctuating levels of consciousness, and hypotonicity, or limpness of skeletal muscles. Dr. Grant went on to explain that NMS is an acute form of exhaustive mania that may be related to a cardiac event due to psychological stress. The processes leading to death are sudden cardiac arrhythmia or respiratory arrest induced by a combination of factors relating to increased oxygen demands and decreased oxygen delivery. In sum, an agitated psychological state—exacerbated by drugs or alcohol abuse and police confrontation, resulting in hyperactivity caused by struggling with restraints—increases oxygen demands on the heart and lungs.

Taking all these factors into account Dr. Grant and I concluded that William Packer's death was accidental, not homicidal. However, case studies show that restraining someone, in a state of mental agitation, prone, or flat, impairs breathing by inhibiting chest wall and diaphragmatic movement. We found no evidence that Packer was asphyxiated. He had died of acute exhaustion. By restraining Packer, his caregivers had unwittingly hastened his demise.

Police and medical caregivers should be warned about the potential lethality of prone restraint in excited, delirious patients. At present, safer methods of controlling violent behavior, such as devices allowing for full restraint while in a seated position, are being developed.

In my final report I concluded:

> Reports of events prior to death seem to indicate some sort of mental disturbance. William

exhibited acute onset of irrational, aggressive, violent behavior with paranoid features, which is referred to in the medical literature as "excited delirium," a rare form of severe mania. Reports in the literature also suggest that such people may die of acute exhaustive mania. Hyperthermia, or heat stroke, is often part of the syndrome. In the absence of a natural or pathologic cause of death we can suggest that the most likely cause of death is Excited Delirium. The mechanism of death appears to be a sudden fatal cardiac dysrhythmia, or respiratory arrest, induced by a combination of factors relating to increased oxygen demands and decreased oxygen delivery. Agitated psychiatric delirium coupled with police confrontation places catecholamine stresses on the heart. Hyperactivity coupled with struggling against restraints increases the oxygen demands of the heart and lungs. The death then is accidental rather than homicidal.

I met with William's brother Ned Packer, and his aunt, Aggie Hinton, to discuss my findings. I could tell that they were still in a state of shock and disbelief at the strange and sudden death of a loved one so far from home. I explained that paranoia refers to an obsessive, unreasonable fear of being harmed by someone or something imagined, not based in reality. Excited delirium refers to a psychotic state during which a person engages in uncontrolled, frenzied movement in an attempt to escape terrifying hallucinations.

Ned was upset; however, the more he understood about what had happened to his brother, the easier it would be for him to find closure, so I continued, "Cardiac dysrhythmia is an abnormal, rapid heart beat which stresses the heart. Aggravating the dysrhythmia are catecholamines, or the hormones adrenaline and nor-adrenaline, which control heart rate. These hormones are secreted in large quantities when a person is frightened, as happened to your brother. You may have heard of the fight and flight response, which causes the heart to speed up and blood pressure to rise as adrenaline is pumped into the blood. This situation continued over a prolonged period of time, putting extreme stress on your brother's heart."

The aunt said that despite explanation and analysis, she still felt that somehow the police and doctors had mistreated her nephew, and that William's death could have been prevented had the embassy sent someone to help him.

I could do little to dispel her suspicions other than to reiterate that we had found no disease process in the organs. Nor was there evidence of traumatic injury. If I had found some proof of physical trauma leading to death—a blow to the head causing cerebral hemorrhage, or a kick in the chest fracturing ribs and puncturing the lungs—it would have provided irrefutable corroboration of wrongdoing and the basis for a lawsuit.

The family persisted in denying that William Packer had suffered from a mental illness, and continued to believe that his death had resulted from mishandling by the authorities. I pointed out that people often hide mental illness. In addition, Mr. Packer was away from home for many years, thus making it easier for him to conceal his condition from them.

My elucidation of a cause of death did not provide a sense of closure to the Packer family: it had not cleared away their confusion, doubt, or anger. In dealing with cases like this, I have come to realize that the bereaved are seeking more than a final medical diagnosis, they are asking philosophical questions about the meaning of life and death, love and loss, for which there are no clear-cut answers.

The Packers accused Consul Delaney of having failed to come to Williams' aid promptly. They pointed out that State Department directives clearly state that, when notified by the local law enforcement officials of the arrest or detention of any U.S. citizen, someone from the embassy should speak to and make an initial visit to the detainee soon afterward, with follow up visits periodically. Although Consul Delaney had received repeated calls from police, medical caregivers, and friends, he made no attempt to visit William.

A semantic battle ensued as to whether "promptly" meant immediately, or as Consul Delaney insisted, "as soon as possible." Although the family could not legally pin the blame on any one individual, they remained convinced that if the consul had come to William's aid, he might not have died. Indeed, it appeared that miscommunication and an unwillingness to take on the responsibility for managing William Packer's mental illness had precipitated his death. Of course, this difficult situation was exacerbated because it occurred in a foreign country.

Many families like the Packers are ill prepared to cope with the discovery that their loved one has a mental illness, yet mental disorders are widespread. An estimated 54 million Americans suffer from some form of mental disorder in a given year. Regrettably, because of the stigma attached to this illness, many individuals may attempt to conceal their condition from friends and family, and do not seek timely and appropriate intervention.

13

A Case of Outrage

The circumstances leading to Ricky Champion's demise proved to be different from any other autopsy I had performed. First, my final anatomical diagnoses uncovered an unusual number of disease processes for an individual who had started out life with an uncomplicated pregnancy, a normal delivery, and as a healthy baby. Yet, from an early age this seemingly well child had developed clinical symptoms of mental retardation, diabetes, seizures, and renal failure. What factors had intervened to damage Ricky Champion's health so drastically and shorten his life span?

Born in a three-roomed, cinder block company house beneath the shadow of the giant factory, let's call it PromTox, Ricky's arrival passed without notice from the world at large. Three decades later, he made news headlines when he caught a strangely deformed fish in Choco Creek that resulted in the State Department of Public Health issuing its first fish consumption advisory. But the spotlight came too late for Ricky, his family, and the residents of the town.

Unbeknown to them, Ricky's illness began with the consumption of produce grown by his maternal grandparents, Booker and Edwina Tyson. The grandparents lived in the valley crammed between Baldwater Mountain and the industrial corridor on the west side of town where the Promtox plant was located. To supplement their income, they kept hogs and cows and grew a variety of vegetables. On his way home from elementary school Ricky often went wading in the factory's drainage ditch running behind his grandparents' house. Sometimes he threw stones at the cows drinking from the ditch just to see them toss their big heads and moo sullenly. To avoid feeding the pigs or weeding the patch of vegetables flourishing in the moist land alongside the channel, he often dawdled in the water. Although his grandparents scolded him for not doing his chores, they worried about their grandson; he was much too puny for a boy his age and tired too quickly. To supplement the family diet, Ricky often went fishing with his grandfather. Even back then he noticed that the fish were sluggish when the creek ran purple, making them easier to snare; sometimes they floated belly-up in the purplish eddies.

These early carefree days of Ricky Champion's childhood were fleeting. Just months before his eighth birthday, Ricky's health began to deteriorate. The first symptom seemed innocuous enough; the boy would raise his hand to ask for permission to go to bathroom much too frequently. Concerned that there was something ailing her student, the teacher asked the district nurse to examine him; the nurse then referred him to Doctor Coombs. When the lab test came back, the doctor called Mrs. Champion to tell her that her boy's problem was grave. He had Type 1 diabetes, and would need daily shots of insulin.

In the summer that Ricky turned eleven, he began suffering from seizures and bouts of rage. Doctor Coombs referred Ricky to a specialist. Unfortunately, the doctor could not find the specific cause of his seizures, but prescribed a medication that reduced their frequency. With each succeeding birthday, Ricky's health took another downward slide. He developed disabilities related to diabetes: severe visual impairment, fatigue, and generalized muscle weakness.

Members of the Champion family, who lived in the town, also came down with serious illnesses. A cousin was diagnosed with colon cancer at a young age. Mrs. Champion's sister developed breast cancer. Others in their neighborhood suffered from a higher than normal incidence of respiratory problems, high blood pressure, arthritis, and kidney diseases, although they were still comparatively young, and did not smoke or drink. The preacher declared that it was God's will, and that they would be rewarded in heaven for their suffering.

It wasn't until the mid 1960s, following a massive fish kill, that Promtox hired a State University biologist, Denzel Ferguson, to conduct studies around its plant. Ferguson and two graduate students packed a tank of bluegill fish into a pickup and headed for the creeks in the vicinity of Promtox. To the dismay of the biologists gathered on the muddy bank that day, within 10 seconds all 25 bluegills lost equilibrium, turned on their sides, and floated lifeless within minutes.

Decades later, Ferguson would testify in court that, "It's like we dunked the fish in battery acid. The bluegills' skins' sloughed off like blood blisters on the bottom of your foot."

In a written report, Ferguson concluded that the problem was the 'extremely toxic' wastewater flowing directly from the Promtox's plant into Snow Creek and from there into Choco Creek, where he noted similar "die-offs." He warned Promtox: "Since this is a surface stream that passes through residential areas, it may represent a potential source of danger to children." He had urged the company to clean up the creek and to stop dumping untreated waste polluted with polychlorinated biphenyls, or PCBs, from their plant. Production of this complex chemical had started as early as 1929, and by the 1940s was being mass-produced for a host of industrial purposes: PCBs were used as coolants in transformers and capacitors, pesticide extenders, dust-reducing agents, as cutting oils and as flame-retardants.

Promtox chose to ignore Ferguson's repeated warnings and did not release the results of his study. At the time, Ferguson was unaware that Promtox officials were meeting behind closed doors to discuss his scientific findings, which they labeled "evil publicity." Despite Promtox' attempt at secrecy, a reporter working for the local newspaper obtained figures from the Food and Drug Administration (FDA) that showed high levels of PCBs in fish from Choco Creek. A memo, which came to light much later, stated that the company successfully averted negative publicity by convincing the reporter to write a "factual" piece emphasizing that there was no cause for public alarm.

Nevertheless, Promtox knew the scientific facts: the plant was the source of thousands of pounds of potentially deadly PCBs. Promtox's own studies found that PCBs caused tumors in rats. The company's tests on rats, chickens, and dogs, showed that PCBs were more toxic than even they had anticipated. And their tests on fish continued to be ominous; in the ensuing years,

Promtox discovered deformed and lethargic fish in the creeks and rivers near the plant with astronomical levels of PCBs. These results were predictable as the plant continued routinely discharging toxic waste into the creek, and to dump toxic waste into open-pit landfills.

Despite these ominous findings, Promtox was not about to give up a lucrative business worth $22 million a year, and continued to squelch or to downplay negative information. The company reworded the scientific findings from 'slightly tumorigenic' to 'does not appear to be carcinogenic.' Throughout the 1980s, Promtox continued to dodge regulators, agreeing only to limited cleanups. Under mounting pressure, the company installed a sump, a carbon bed, and a new limestone pit to trap PCBs. However, these measures were not enough to prevent people from ingesting the dangerous chemical in the food chain. At least $1 billion in additional pollution controls were necessary to effectively prevent contamination of the water and soil.

Finally in the 1990s, Promtox's campaign to downgrade the dangers of PCBs became a hot topic in the national media. Members of Congress began calling for hearings. Fearing that it could be forced to shut down certain plants if government regulators discovered the amount of PCBs spewing into the river, company officials formed an ad hoc committee, which put several options on the table. One committee proposed that they 'sell the hell out of the product as long as it was possible to do so.' Another recommended that they phase out the product, but only after they had developed an alternative. A third committee advised that they reduce PCBs discharge only to the legal minimum. All agreed that there was no benefit to a unilateral crackdown on Promtox's PCBs when its customers were still dumping it wholesale. One of its biggest customers urged Promtox to keep producing PCBs because it helped prevent power outages and, they claimed, the environmental threat had still to be proven.

Concerned about possible legal action, Promtox made the decision to inform the State Water Improvement Commission that PCBs were entering Snow Creek. To limit the damage, Promtox's executives assured the commission that everything was under control. In a memo, the head of the commission advised Promtox: Give no statements or publications that would bring the situation to the public's attention. If word leaked out, the state would be forced to ban fishing in Choco Creek, a popular recreational lake downstream.

While the machinations between Promtox and the state water improvement commission continued, Ricky and the folks in the town kept on swimming in the creeks, eating fish caught there, and allowing their livestock to drink the water. While many were concerned about Promtox dumping its waste into their creeks and waterways, they needed the jobs provided by the company.

Then in 1993, Ricky Champion caught a bizarrely deformed largemouth bass in Choco Creek. By that time he knew enough to report it to a newsman working for the local paper. The newsman tipped off a biologist at the nearby university. The biologist's tests measured extremely high levels of PCBs in the fish. The newsman revealed the ominous findings in the local paper, this time without putting a positive spin on them. For the first time, the state issued advisories against eating fish caught in the area—almost thirty years after Promtox learned about those bluegills sloughing off their skins as if dunked in battery acid.

Stories, like the smell of rotten-eggs from Promtox when a steady wind blew, began to spread around the town. One resident swore that the soles of his boots burnt off after walking over the Promtox landfill. Bernice Champion, Ricky's mother, said that her dogs had died after drinking from the drainage ditch behind her parents' home. Alarmed residents began holding meetings to investigate the high number of people living near the creek suffering from cancer.

Three years later, residents hired Nathan Bork, an attorney, with a law firm known for winning environmental cases. On behalf of the residents, the firm filed charges against Promtox in the state court. The lawsuits uncovered a voluminous paper trail, revealing details of secret corporate machinations in the era before strict environmental regulations and right-to-know laws. There were documents dating as far back as the 1930s that exposed actions with life-threatening consequences for the residents of the town. Promtox could no longer hide the fact that for decades it had discharged unfiltered and untreated PCB waste directly into streams, or dumped it in landfills around town. Promtox employees had carried the toxic chemical home on their work clothes.

Bernice Champion was the star witness for the plaintiffs. She related how years before, a man from Promtox had knocked on her door and declared that her hogs were trespassing on company property. He ordered her to get the hogs off their property within twenty-four hours. As there was no place for hogs in her small yard, Mrs. Champion didn't know where to turn. She thought of calling her brother to come and slaughter the hogs, but where could she find a crew to cut, clean and freeze the meat before it went bad? She was sitting on her porch crying, when the employee from Promtox returned with an offer to buy the hogs for $25 a head, plus a pint of white corn liquor. Mrs. Champion said that she didn't drink, but Christmas was coming and she was short on cash, so she agreed to the deal. In court that day, Mrs. Champion learned, for the first time, about Promtox's clandestine research on hogs. Thirty years earlier, the company had dissected hogs from the area she lived in, and found PCB levels as high as 19,000 parts per million—more than 90,000 times the legal maximum in some states today.

Brandishing her fist in the air she hissed, "We ate them hogs and it made us sick to death!"

After years of legal wrangling, Promtox settled the class action for about $40 million. The Champions got just $32,000. But no amount of money could restore Ricky's health. By this time he had developed coronary artery and heart disease, both complications of diabetes. His parents reluctantly placed Ricky in a nursing home.

Shortly after that, the Champion's neighborhood was declared a public health hazard. Promtox then launched a program to buy and raze homes in the polluted area. As incentives, they offered the residents early sign-up bonuses and moving expenses. Like many others, the Champions could not afford to buy a new home with the amount Promtox offered. After over 100 PCB-tainted homes and small businesses were demolished. The few remaining residents moved away, leaving behind abandoned houses, lots choked with weeds, and streets piled with trash.

Just before his fortieth birthday, Ricky succumbed to the host of illnesses that had plagued him for years. The family retained Nathan Bork to file a suit on their son's behalf. Bork explained that Ricky would serve as the test case to prove that PCBs not only affected health adversely; the ingestion of the chemical could ultimately result in death. The attorney warned the

Champions that it would not be easy, because the company's lawyers would do everything in their power to cast doubt that PCBs were a direct cause of illness and death. They would need to call in expert researchers in the field, and to perform an autopsy on Ricky in order to substantiate their claim.

Upon the request of the lawyers, for both the plaintiffs and defendants, I performed an autopsy. The deceased was markedly underweight with visible skeletal bones on the chest and limbs. Upon the chest I observed that the pericardium, or covering of the heart, was distended like a balloon. The cavity of the sac surrounding the heart was filled with yellowish-green, viscous pus; normally this cavity contains only a few centimeters of watery fluid. I removed the heart from the cavity, noting that the normally smooth and shiny surface had become dull with adherent yellow mucoid, or mucus-like material, sticking to the surface.

I removed and sliced the lungs in half to reveal numerous cavities filled with the same thick pus, indicating pulmonary abscesses. The surrounding lung tissue was beefy, red and solid. I noted that the liver was enlarged, and upon dissection, saw that the normally uniform, reddish brown surface had become speckled with little red dots, and the liver tissue was pale yellow, giving it the speckled appearance of a fresh nutmeg. The spleen, normally rubbery, had become soft and mushy, and crumbled into irregular pieces when I sliced it with a scalpel. The kidneys had a very irregular cobblestone appearance, when they should normally be smooth and shiny. The urinary bladder was full of greenish pus, with a red and thickened lining.

I harvested samples of the liver, pancreas, kidney and brain by slicing the tissue into squares, about one-eighth inch thick, with a scalpel and then placing them in fixative for processing into slides to be viewed under the microscope. I labeled and placed them in separate containers and submitted them to a lab for analysis of the PCB isomers (two or more substances composed of the same elements but with different arrangements of atoms). The test results showed that PCB isomers were present in significant concentrations in Ricky's liver and kidneys. Lesser amounts were present in the brain tissue. PCB isomers were thus present in his vital organs.

In the conclusion to my autopsy report, I stated that:

The immediate cause of death is acute pericarditis and acute bronchopneumonia. PCB intoxication is long standing, resulting in major damage and loss of function of the liver, pancreas, kidneys and brain. This is evidenced clinically by early onset of diabetes mellitus, renal failure, neurological symptoms, emaciation and immobility. The multi organ damage also results in the inability to fight off infection by compromising the immune system, thus contributing to the findings of the cause of death.

My findings corroborated numerous epidemiological studies, which demonstrated an association between PCB's, and diabetes and liver problems.

After months of testimony, a jury reached a decision to hold Promtox and the company representing its chemical division, liable on six counts: negligence, nuisance, suppression of the truth, trespass, wantonness, and outrage. The claim of outrage, under this particular state's law, is rarely won because it requires that the plaintiff prove conduct "so outrageous in character and extreme in degree as to go beyond all possible bounds of decency so as to be regarded as atrocious and utterly intolerable in a civilized society."

When the verdict was issued in their favor, the Champions invited relatives and friends to a picnic by the creek where Ricky had once loved to fish, to sing, and to pray. Everyone brought something good to eat, but not a single homegrown vegetable because the Environmental Protection Agency found that the dirt in their gardens had high levels of PCBs.

The old plant off Promtox Road had stopped the actual manufacturing of PCBs in the 1970s, but Promtox's legacy of toxic pollution remains as deeply embedded in the town's psyche as in its red clay soil. PCBs do not degrade. They persist in the environment, accumulate in humans and wildlife, and are transported worldwide by air and water. In addition, there are leakage of PCBs from transformers and capacitors still in use. Because they bio-accumulate (build up in fatty tissues over time), it is likely to take many years for the full effect to be realized. Although EPA and the World Health Organization classify PCBs as "probable carcinogens," the company has opposed proposals for comprehensive clean up and in-depth health studies as unnecessary.

Far from the national spotlight, the battle still rages In Ricky's town, and the wrongdoings of the past are still being visited upon the residents. Although Promtox and its corporate successors spent $40 million on cleanup efforts, they spent millions more on hiring lawyers to fight legal settlements. New lawsuits by the town's residents continue to be scheduled for trial.

The events preceding Ricky Champion's slow and painful demise left me dismayed and outraged that my fellow human beings could so easily and unwittingly become hapless victims of individual and corporate avarice. In my opinion, it is imperative that we all work together to abate environmental pollution that adversely affects public health.

14

The Exhumation of Wiley Root

I am rarely called upon to autopsy the remains of an exhumed corpse. More recently, however, as a result of improved DNA testing, the number of exhumations has risen. To unearth evidence of a crime the famous and infamous have been exhumed for DNA tests, among them the outlaw Jesse James, President Zachary Taylor, the civil rights leader, Medgar Evers, and the assassin Lee Harvey Oswald. The most common reason, however, for disinterring a corpse is to obtain DNA to settle paternity suits as occurred between Yvonne Jenkins and the children of Wiley Root, the man she claimed to be her father.

The circumstances surrounding the exhumation of eighty-four-year-old Wiley Root started with a gruesome car crash. Root died in the accident, while his son Albert, riding in the passenger seat, survived with minor injuries. From his hospital bed just hours after the accident, Albert described the seconds preceding the crash to Joe Selig, a young news reporter. He recalled hearing a loud bang as the front tires blew and the SUV swerved wildly across the road. Next thing he knew the car flipped three times and he found himself trapped upside down by the air bag.

His suspicions aroused, the reporter ferreted out several articles asserting that five years ago, Elasdeluxe had found a defect in their tires, which company engineers labeled "alarming." In response the engineers had changed the design to strengthen the tires, but Elasdeluxe chose not to notify the federal government or to recall the millions of tires already on the road. The defective tires were still being sold under numerous names.

Once he became aware of the situation, Albert Root retained an attorney. Mr. Paul Morris, to a file a claim against Elasdeluxe. In addition, Albert petitioned the court to suspend probating the late Mr. Wiley Root's will, pending the outcome of the suit.

Weeks after Wiley Root's funeral, an article about the Root's suit against Elasdeluxe appeared in the local newspaper with Jo Selig's byline. The next day, a woman by the name of

Yvonne Jenkins came forward to claim that she was the daughter of the late Wiley Root, and therefore entitled to her share of any settlement made by Elasdeluxe. Mrs. Jenkins told the three Root children that her mother had given birth to her at sixteen. Wiley Root, whom she called Daddy, had visited them regularly. She looked forward to him coming because he always brought a treat or a toy. Six years ago, before her mother passed on, she told her daughter that she had three half siblings living in the town. Mrs. Jenkins said that she had not contacted her three siblings then because she did not want to cause trouble. However, since Wiley Root's will stipulated that his estate should be divided equally between his children, as his daughter she was entitled to her share.

The Root children—Albert, Lottie and Caroline—were outraged. They felt that Mrs. Jenkins was nothing but a shameless imposter. They warned her that they wanted nothing to do with her. As a result, she retained Sam Bailey as her lawyer. Bailey advised Mrs. Jenkins that if she went before the probate judge claiming that she was a legitimate heir, the judge would ask for evidence to prove her claim. Bailey explained that if her DNA matched Wiley Root's DNA, then it would prove that she was his daughter. Although Root would have to be exhumed, testing could be performed on virtually any remaining body part like a bone or a tooth. Bailey said that Mrs. Jenkins would need to apply to the state's attorney general for permission to exhume the body.

However, if the probate judge determined that there was good cause, he would grant her request for exhumation and for reburial without the need for the attorney general.

On behalf of Mrs. Jenkins, Bailey, her attorney, contracted me to obtain the necessary samples from Willey Root, if the exhumation was allowed. I would send these to a lab specializing in DNA testing, whose results would hold up in a court of law. Since the disinterment of a corpse is an exceedingly delicate process, I do not undertake it lightly. I first obtained the lawyer's assurance that he would get legal permission from all interested parties; that the grave would be properly identified; that workers would take proper protective health measures; and that arrangements would be made to mechanically excavate the site. The casket would be transferred to the funeral home where I could collect the necessary specimens.

Two weeks later, I met Mrs. Jenkins and Mr. Bailey at the funeral home, where Wiley Root's casket sat on a table. I noticed that the casket, constructed of dark wood, had fittings with the mat finish of pewter rather than the gleam of stainless steel. The funeral director stepped forward and removed a plastic box from a compartment in the lid of the coffin.

"The keys are kept here for just such occasions as these," he said, withdrawing a key.

As he turned the key in the lock it made a grating sound of metal against metal. The director tried several times to open the lock then declared that the locking mechanism was frozen. He thought that the long, spiral screw of the lock seemed to have rusted out. The only way to open it was to take a sledgehammer to the locks. He warned, however, that he would not break the locks without a replacement casket. Mrs. Jenkins replied that she did not have the money to do pay for a new casket. I pointed out that if I did not collect the tissue for DNA testing, all the trouble and expense of exhuming Mr. Root would be to no avail. The director agreed, complaining that the locks were supposed to be made of stainless steel and should not have rusted. I asked if the casket manufacturer issued a warranty on the locks, whereupon Mr. Bailey advised the director to call the casket manufacturer to tell him that their product had failed. It took several phone calls to ascertain that Mr. Root's casket had a limited 5-year warranty. Since Mr. Root was interred less than a year ago, the manufacturer agreed to replace the casket.

While the funeral director used a sledgehammer to break the locks and open the casket, Mrs. Jenkins waited anxiously in the parlor with the customary crowded arrangements of silk flowers set on faux gold pedestals, plush wine-colored carpet, and chairs upholstered in artificial blue velvet.

Inside the coffin I found the embalmed body of Willy

Root in a fair state of preservation. Using the tools of my trade—scalpel, forceps and bone saw—I removed samples of skin, muscles, and bone, and placed them in sealed plastic bags. I labeled each bag with the name, date, time of collection, and the anatomical site from which tissue had been removed. I then collected a blood sample from Pricilla Jenkins, to be mailed to the qualified lab along with the tissue samples.

The results arrived about two weeks later. The DNA of Yvonne Jenkins and Wiley Roots matched with ninety-percent certainty.

When the Roots' case against Elasdeluxe came to trial, their attorney, Paul Morris, argued that Wiley Root died of injuries sustained when the tire treads on the vehicle he was driving peeled away, causing the vehicle to roll over. His investigations proved that the rubber compound used in the Elasdeluxe tires did not adhere properly to the brass coating of the steel belt, causing the treads to come apart. Morris alleged that Elasdeluxe provided insufficient warning to the public about this defect and knowingly sold a malfunctioning tire.

Elasdeluxe's lawyers countered that the tires on Wiley Root's SUV were five years old. They argued that although the tires had been repaired just three days before the accident, the repair shop was to blame because the tires should never have been put back on the vehicle. Elasdeluxe's lawyers asserted that poorly repaired punctures, even on the safest tires, cause tire treads to separate.

The jury did not accept the arguments put forward by Elasdeluxe. They agreed that there should have been adequate warnings posted about the defective tires. The jury awarded $4.7 million to the Root children.

Subsequently, a judge ruled that Mrs. Jenkins was entitled to her share of the settlement. If any one dared to accuse her of greed, she told them in no uncertain terms that her three young children should not have to pay for the sins of their grandparents.

This was a case where science supplied the answers, enabling justice to be served. Is DNA testing absolutely reliable? It is, but there is a growing problem in this burgeoning field. Lab workers collecting the DNA samples and performing the analysis can make mistakes. Consequently, although DNA is reliable as a definitive science, the technicians reading and analyzing the samples may become the source of inaccurate results.

Future Diagnosis

After reading these case histories, I hope that the reader will recognize that the autopsy remains the benchmark for making the decisive final diagnosis. Knowledge gleaned at autopsy has been integral to understanding the disease process, to developing new therapies and to evaluating the precision of new diagnostic technologies, including modern imaging techniques. Despite advances in technology, which physicians have come to depend on, examination of the organs of the body macroscopically and microscopically reveals pathology that could not otherwise be detected. In addition, the autopsy is a valuable tool for providing undergraduate and graduate medical students with a scientific method of identifying and understanding the pathogenesis, or development and causes of disease. The findings at autopsy can and should improve the physician's ability to make an accurate clinical diagnosis. In sum, the autopsy provides an important tool for monitoring the quality of medical care

Too often overlooked is the comfort that the findings of the autopsy provide to family and friends during the grieving period. My own experience, supported by research, has convinced me that understanding the cause of death helps survivors resolve their feelings of guilt about whether their loved ones received proper and adequate care before their demise.

Despite all the benefits that the autopsy can provide, the number performed in the US has markedly declined. There are several reasons for this. First, there is no monetary incentive for the hospital pathologist. The principal agency accrediting hospitals—The Joint Commission on the Accreditation of Healthcare Organizations, or JCAHO—eliminated a requirement for a minimal autopsy rate many years ago. Medicare stopped paying directly for autopsies in 1986; since Medicare does not reimburse, the hospital must bear the cost, and the pathologist perform the autopsy as a free service. As a result, almost all medical schools have reduced or eliminated the teaching of autopsy pathology; worse yet, many young physicians have never witnessed an autopsy. In addition, hospital pathologists themselves are given few incentives for doing an autopsy. The pathologist's primary responsibilities are surgical pathology, running the clinical laboratory, and interpreting biopsies and organ resections for living people. Medical autopsies take several hours, while getting results out to other clinicians for his patients is a priority; doctors expect results within 24 hours of the procedure.

Yet another cause for the decline in autopsies is a lack of recognition of the significance of the autopsy among doctors themselves. Many clinicians hold the mistaken belief that modern technology provides all that is required for accurate diagnosis, and because of their limited exposure to cadavers in anatomy class and to autopsy procedures, the doctor may feel that nothing new can be gleaned from the autopsy. As a result, many physicians do not discuss the need for autopsies with family members or advise them that they can request the autopsy with the next-of-kin signing an authorization.

Finally, but not foremost, doctors may fear lawsuits if autopsies uncover something they missed.

Compounding this unfortunate situation, the teaching of the autopsy procedure during residency training is declining, although the College of American Pathologists still recognizes the value of the autopsy and encourages its use. There is no hard data currently available about the quality of the autopsies performed today; however, my own experience, and that of some colleagues, indicates that missed diagnoses are increasing in number at the autopsy table due to lack of training at medical schools. Similarly, I have the uneasy perception that the ability of pathology residents to evaluate pathology in surgical specimens may have declined. Exacerbating the situation, some of the newer hospitals are being built without morgues, or existent morgues have been converted to storage areas.

In closing, I would strongly recommend that the autopsy be maintained as a valuable procedure for improving the overall standard of medical care, and that insurance companies or other providers reimburse the costs for this procedure, where appropriate, thus making it more accessible.

As my own colleagues retire, I wonder who will be assigned to perform autopsies and whether he or she will know how to do them competently. The autopsy is for me, and for other physicians, a privileged opportunity to advance medical knowledge and to contribute to the well being of society as a whole.

ABOUT THE AUTHOR

Boris Datnow M.D. FCAP, has practiced pathology for over forty years. During this period he performed autopsies, from which he carefully selected cases for this book. Dr. Datnow was awarded a Post-Doctoral Fellowship from the National Academy of Sciences and the National Research Council to conduct research at the Ames Research Center in Moffett Field, California. After completing a residency in Clinical and Anatomic Pathology at the Mayo Clinic Graduate School of Medicine in Rochester, Minnesota, he was elected a Fellow of the American Board of Pathology. He continues his work as a pathologist to the present time.

CONTRIBUTOR

Claire Datnow MA, has published numerous works of fiction and nonfiction. She taught creative writing to gifted and talented students. *Edwin Hubble: Discoverer of Galaxies*, and *American Science Fiction and Fantasy Writers* are some of her publications for young adults. Born in South Africa, she immigrated to the United States in 1965 with her husband Boris Datnow. Claire has received numerous scholarships and grants including a Beeson Samford University Writing Project fellowship, a Folk Life Grant from the Alabama Arts Council, and a Fulbright Memorial Fund Teacher scholarship to travel to Japan.

Proof

Made in the USA